CATCHING THE WAVE:

A History of the University of California, San Diego

School of Medicine

David N. Bailey, M.D.

Distinguished Research Professor of Pathology and Pharmacy

University of California, San Diego

9500 Gilman Drive

La Jolla, California 92093 – 0612

(dnbailey@ucsd.edu; 858: 822-5551)

(2018 Update)

(Author's Note: A complimentary Powerpoint PDF file of this history with pictures is available by contacting the author at the e-mail address shown above).

Dedication

This book is dedicated to the University of California, San Diego School of Medicine faculty, who

are the reason the school has achieved its prominence.

Acknowledgements

The author thanks Marilyn G. Farquhar, Distinguished Professor and Founding Chair of the UC San Diego Department of Cellular and Molecular Medicine, for inspiring and encouraging me to write this history. I also thank John Alksne, Richard C. Atkinson, Edward Dennis, Richard Gallo, Gabriel Haddad, Jess Mandel, Gerard Manecke, Gary Matthews, Charles Nager, Maria Randerson, Andrew L. Ries, Doris Trauner, and Rebecca Woolston for providing information that was not readily available through UC San Diego archival material. I am grateful to John Alksne, Elizabeth Barrett-Connor, Marilyn G. Farquhar, Gordon Gill, Joan Heller-Brown, Roger Meyer, Thomas Moore, William Nyhan, Marshall Orloff, Andrew L. Ries, Palmer Taylor, and John West for sharing their personal insights about factors contributing to the rapid rise to prominence of the UC San Diego School of Medicine.

David N. Bailey

Contents

Chapter 1

Introduction

Although I have lived in La Jolla, California for 40 years I have never surfed. However, I understand that surfing requires extraordinary skill, patience, coordination, a good sense of timing, and plain old good luck. The elements have to just right in order to catch the wave and to ride it successfully. In many ways this metaphor applies to the UC San Diego School of Medicine, which caught the wave early on and has ridden it successfully for many years thus far.

Expanding upon this metaphor, ironically, UC San Diego, located next to the Pacific Ocean, has been rated one of the nation's best schools for surfing [1]. Its School of Medicine by any measure has risen to prominence quickly since its founding about 50 years ago. As of this writing, 57 UC San Diego faculty members (current and emeritus) are members of the National Academy of Medicine [2]. Sixteen of the UC San Diego members of the National Academy of Sciences have appointments in the school of medicine [3]. Six Nobel laureates have been affiliated with the school of medicine with one being a dean [4]. The school is one of the top ten medical schools in the nation with the lowest acceptance (most competitive) rates for students [5], and it is ranked among the top 20 best global universities for clinical medicine [6]. It has consistently been rated by *US News and World Report* within the top 20 United States medical schools when ranked by both research and primary care [7]. Furthermore, its health system has been consistently ranked as the top system in San Diego by the *US News and World Report's Best Hospitals*, has been named among the "100 Great Hospitals in America" by *Becker's Hospital Review*, and has been listed as one of the nation's "Top 100 Hospitals" by

Truven Health [8]. The UC San Diego Health System has San Diego's only regional burn center, the region's first level 1 trauma center, one of the first five accredited comprehensive stroke centers in the nation, and one of only 47 designated comprehensive cancer centers in the nation [9].

Since joining the UC San Diego School of Medicine faculty in 1977 I have been blessed with the opportunity of serving as a department chair (14 years); an interim vice chancellor for health sciences and dean of the school of medicine twice; and deputy vice chancellor for health sciences, deputy dean, and dean for faculty and student matters (6 years). These positions have provided me with the opportunity of experiencing first-hand the remarkable rise to prominence of the institution. That said, I feel "duty-bound" to write the story and to investigate the factors ("the secrets to success") that led to its rapid ascent.

Shortly after embarking on writing this history I realized that I was faced with a dilemma, namely that the project was sufficiently large that it could easily be overwhelmed with minute facts that could obscure its major purpose: to outline the evolution of the school in enough detail as to determine the factors most responsible for its rapid ascent. On the other hand, failure to provide enough detail could result in producing merely a cursory overview of the school. Accordingly, I have tried to achieve an appropriate balance between these two extremes. Of necessity, that has meant that I have neither provided mention of every major player or event in the school's history nor provided exquisite detail about those people and events that are covered. Of particular note is the fact that I have not profiled the rich developmental history of individual academic departments since, given the magnitude of accomplishments in the departments, each is worthy of a book unto itself! Instead, I have woven departments and their chairs into the overall story as they pertain to the school and its development. Similarly, I have not covered details about many of the talented associate deans and the numerous staff who have played significant roles in the development of the school. To those readers who may be offended by these omissions, I offer my apology.

David N. Bailey

La Jolla, California

July 16, 2017

References

1. C. Clark: UC San Diego Rides Wave of Recognition as Top Surfing School, February 21, 2013.
   (http://UCSDnews.UCSD.edu/feature/uc_san_diego_rides_wave_of_recognition_as_top_surfing_school)
2. M. Brubaker: Two UC San Diego Researchers Elected to National Academy of Medicine. UC San Diego Health News Release, October 17, 2016
   (https://health.ucsd.edu/news/releases/pages/2016-10-17-anderson-and-sallis-elected-to-national-academy-of-medicine)
3. Membership directory, National Academy of Sciences
   (http://www.nasonline.org/member-directory/)
4. University of California Nobel Laureates
   (http://nobel.universityofcalifornia.edu/list.html)
5. *US News and World Report* 2017: 10 Medical Schools with the Lowest Acceptance Rates
   (http://www.usnews.com/education/best-graduate-schools/the-short-list-grad-school/articles/2016-03-17/10-medical-schools-with-the-lowest-acceptance-rates)
6. *US News and World Report Best Global Universities for Clinical Medicine* 2017
   (https://www.usnews.com/education/best-global-universities/clinical-medicine?page=2)
7. *US News and World Report 2017* (https://www.usnews.com/best-graduate-schools/top-medical-schools)
8. UC San Diego Health Awards & Achievements
   (https://health.ucsd.edu/about/pages/awards-achievements.aspx)
9. At a Glance: UC San Diego Health
   (https://health.ucsd.edu/about/documents/overview.pdf)

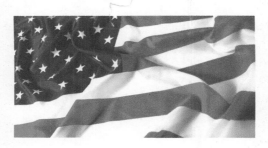

Today

Today

Chapter 2

Starting From Scratch: Thinking Out of the Box

(1958 – 1972)

The seeds for this incredible story were sown in 1958 when the San Diego County Hospital Committee asked the Regents of the University of California (UC) to consider establishment of a medical school in San Diego, offering use of the county hospital for clinical teaching. At that time the UC system had only two schools of medicine (UC Los Angeles and at UC San Francisco).

While there were 175 physicians for every 100,000 people in California, only one in three applying for a California medical license had received medical education in California [1]. UC President Robert Sproul rejected the proposal due to the poor condition of the aging three-story hospital building, constructed in 1904 and residing in Hillcrest. After considerable lobbying of the legislature by the hospital committee, UC President Clark Kerr, who followed Sproul, agreed to reconsider it [2]. Subsequently in 1961 State of California Governor Edmund ("Pat") Brown declared that the next UC medical school would be built in San Diego next to a planned new county hospital.

In 1962 the UC Regents approved establishment of a medical school in San Diego, and the County of San Diego offered more than 40 acres if UC would agree to operate the new hospital [3]. The agreed upon cost for the medical school was $54 million. The school was to provide "broad-gauged and high-quality education of physicians for service" with 30 students to be enrolled as early as 1964 and with teaching to occur at the county hospital until a basic science building could be constructed on the UC San Diego campus in La Jolla. There was basic disagreement between those who desired to create a school with emphasis on research (based on campus) (as originally proposed to the UC Regents by President Kerr) and those who desired to create a school with emphasis on practice (based near the county hospital) (as championed by community practitioners). The UC Regents plans at that time included a 250-bed hospital and clinical research building on the La Jolla campus [2]. The then UC San Diego Chancellor Herbert York stated that "At UCSD we desire to develop a school which meets the needs of modern medical science, which recognizes the best possible fusion between basic science and applied medicine, and which might pioneer some reforms in the structure of medical schools" [4].

The new 600-bed county hospital was completed in 1963 at a cost of $11.5 million for both the building and equipment, with the University subsequently assuming lease of the facility in 1966 as its primary clinical teaching site. Notably the entire inpatient area was opened to private patients of the teaching staff, and the separate private patient area was discontinued. Furthermore, clinical laboratory, radioisotope laboratory, diagnostic radiology, and the cobalt radiation therapy unit were also opened for referral by all San Diego physicians. The University planned to spend $10 million over three to five years to update the facility with a local campaign to raise $1 million for those projects that neither the state nor federal government would fund. Plans included a cardiac intensive care unit, dialysis unit, transplant unit, electroencephalography suite, gift shop, operating room equipment, surgery research laboratory equipment, a staff dining room, and a seminar room. Notable deficiencies at the time included teaching space, inadequate faculty offices and research space, and intensive care unit space [3, 5, 6].

After a national search, on January 1, 1964, Joseph Stokes III was appointed the first dean of the UC San Diego School of Medicine at age 39. Dr. Stokes was a distinguished internist and cardiovascular epidemiologist who had received his Doctor of Medicine degree from Harvard and had completed his internship at Johns Hopkins followed by two years of fellowship in preventive medicine at the Massachusetts General Hospital. For the two years prior to his appointment he had been special consultant for medical education planning at Queens Hospital and University of Hawaii, Honolulu [7].

At the time of appointment of Joseph Stokes as dean it was envisioned that the basic science portion of the medical school curriculum would be taught by the campus departments. This vision was articulated by David Bonner, the chair of the Department of Biology, who stated that "there is no such thing as basic versus applied science; there is only good or bad science" [8]. According to the "Bonner Plan," via a process called "interdigitation," campus departments would be given state FTEs (state-funded lines) by the medical school for teaching. With only technical oversight by Dean Stokes, the so-called "participating departments" on campus could hire whomever they wished with space being provided in the new medical school basic science building, albeit that the faculty would not have to work there and would not even necessarily have to be the ones teaching the medical school classes! The then Chancellor John Galbraith championed this view, envisioning a medical school with no basic science departments at all and with entrance requirements being the same as those for biology graduate students [2]. First-year courses in cellular biology, biochemistry, physiology, biophysics, biomathematics, bioengineering, psychology, medical ecology, and humanities would be taught by the campus departments [9]. Thus, one group of science departments would provide the education for all graduate students, be they Ph.D. or M.D. [8].

Shortly after his appointment Dean Stokes boasted that the new school hopes to attract medical scholars who are "able and willing to innovate, investigate, and educate. The academic environment here is such that it should attract the right kind of scholar. We want UCSD School of Medicine to be tied together by more than just a common parking problem. Any school is fundamentally a collection of scholars and a medical school is no different. So greatly has scientific investigation advanced medicine that today's generation of doctors can hardly speak to the doctors of a generation ago. The research output of the medical school is every bit as important as the number of students who are graduated" [4].

During the months following Dean Stokes arrival the campus revised the plan for the school of medicine with an amended price tag of $122.3 million! President Kerr refused to submit this drastic revision to the UC Regents, ultimately leading to the resignation of Chancellor Galbraith. Instead, Kerr recommended a $58.3 million plan that included a campus hospital, but the UC Regents opted for use of the Hillcrest facility instead, thereby altering their original 1962 decision for a campus hospital. In September 1966 groundbreaking occurred for the $15.5 million school of medicine basic science building. Just two days later and shortly before his resignation as Chancellor, Galbraith relieved Stokes of his deanship after Stokes tried to force private practitioners to pool their income into the medical school teaching and research fund, nearly causing a revolt among community physicians [2]. Upon stepping down as dean, Stokes became chair of the newly created Department of Preventive Medicine [10]. Galbraith then appointed Robert Tschirgi, UC San Diego Vice Chancellor for Academic Affairs, as Acting Dean [2].

Not surprisingly, the removal of Dean Stokes after only 2.5 years caused postponement of the entry date for the first students to 1968. After a protracted search for the second dean, Clifford Grobstein, Ph.D., an internationally renowned developmental biology and National Academy of Sciences member who had been recruited to UC San Diego in 1965 to succeed David Bonner as Professor and Chair of the Department of Biology, was appointed Vice Chancellor for Medicine and Biological Sciences and Dean of the School of Medicine on May 18, 1967 [2, 11]. Interestingly, Grobstein had served as chair of the committee that had developed the first-year medical school curriculum. Like David Bonner, Grobstein articulated interest in developing a new school with a different approach to medical education, namely "that of interdigitation of the general campus and the medical school departments" [9]. Grobstein's outstanding scientific credentials, his decisiveness and ability to act, his ability to be fair (even when it was not in his own interest), and his emphasis on dialog rather than confrontation were hallmarks of his administrative expertise. Furthermore, under his leadership, UC San Diego School of Medicine became a national leader in attracting minority and women candidates [12].

In 1968, with the new vice chancellor/dean in place, the fledgling school of medicine finally matriculated its first class of 47 students from more than 1,000 applicants: 30 from California, 15 from other states, and 2 from other countries with 39 men and 8 women [2]. Students who were state of California residents paid $609 in fees while out-of-state students paid $1,560. Total costs for in-state residents (including living expenses, books, incidentals, and housing) were $2,539 [Maria Randerson, personal communication and research, May 17, 2017].

Robert Hamburger, one of the school's founding faculty, characterized the first students as "daring people" who came to a medical school with no history [13]. The basic science thrust of the school was apparent from the start when the first lecture was given by Nobel laureate Linus Pauling. Also, early on, campus graduate students sat in classes with the medical students. However, this was gradually discontinued because graduate students were not allowed to do their dissertation research in the medical school [13]. If performance on standardized examinations is any indication of a successful curriculum, then this approach to teaching the basic sciences was a success because the school's second class of 48 students placed first in the nation on the 1971 Part I National Board of Medical Examiner's Examination (8,000 students from 81 medical schools participated in that examination) [14].

Regrettably the basic science building, funded by the State of California, the Public Health Service, and the National Institutes of Health, was only partially completed when the initial students arrived but was finished within their first year [15, 16]. Additional plans at that time called for construction of a clinical science building and a Veterans Affairs hospital by 1970. In reality, ground-breaking for the $30 million, 800-bed Veterans Affairs hospital occurred in 1969 with the facility opening in 1972 [3]. Interestingly, a 350-bed campus hospital was again included in planning for two years hence [17], but plans for both the clinical science building and the campus hospital were subsequently scuttled due to shortfalls in the state budget [2]. Thus, for the foreseeable future, the school of medicine would have a completely split campus with pre-clinical education being based in La Jolla and clinical training occurring 13 miles away in Hillcrest. This separation was indeed problematic for many faculty, who had their research laboratories and offices on the La Jolla campus while their clinical teaching was in Hillcrest. For other faculty, who were based on only one of the two campuses, this geographical separation sometimes led to philosophical separation since, admittedly, faculty based on the La Jolla campus frequently had better offices and laboratories [David N. Bailey, personal recollections and research].

By the time of arrival of the first medical students in 1968 nine departments were under development in the school of medicine: community medicine, medicine, neurosciences (which included neurology), obstetrics-gynecology (later to become reproductive medicine), pathology, pediatrics, psychiatry, radiology, and surgery [18]. Given that the basic sciences were taught by the campus departments, such departments were not established in the school of medicine.

By 1972, under the leadership of Vice Chancellor and Dean Grobstein, the school of medicine had grown to 235 students, 332 interns and residents, and 75 postdoctoral fellows and graduate students [2]. Having launched the school and having seen the its inaugural class graduate, Grobstein then resigned and returned to Biology, one year later becoming the UC San Diego Vice Chancellor for University Relations [19]. In his June 11, 1972, commencement remarks to the charter class before he stepped down as dean, Grobstein observed that "Modern medicine is a composite, an amalgam of three ingredients – understanding, skill and compassion. Alone, understanding may have no practical consequence, skill alone can quickly be uncoupled from purpose and direction, compassion alone can degenerate into helpless sympathy or, worse, sentimentality. It is only the amalgam out of which effective health care can be constructed" [20].

Robert Hamburger described the young school as having "zero-activation energy" in that it was able to get more done in less time. He attributed the tremendous faculty productivity to the fact that faculty recruits were able to take free time based upon their work schedule and not on the weather since the weather was always nice in La Jolla. He also noted that new recruits were "offered the moon" in the sense that they were given the freedom to do what they wanted. In addition, if any idea was good, it was generally funded regardless of its expense (programs, buildings, etc.). According to Hamburger, these factors contributed to UC San Diego School of Medicine being a "fantastic upstart"! [21].

References

1. Medical School Plans Hinge on Proposition 1, Stokes Says, October 20, 1964, University Communications & Public Relations Materials: News Releases. Special Collections & Archives, UC San Diego Library.
2. N.A. Anderson. An Improbable Venture: A History of the University of California, San Diego. The UCSD Press, La Jolla, California, 1993, pp 153-180.
3. UC San Diego Health: About Us – Our History (https://health.ucsd.edu/about/pages/history.aspx)
4. Medical School Development, March 9, 1964, University Communications & Public Relations Materials: News Releases. Special Collections & Archives, UC San Diego Library.
5. University Hospital Opens Inpatient Area, January 5, 1967, University Communications & Public Relations Materials: News Releases. Special Collections & Archives, UC San Diego Library.
6. UCSD To Spend $10 Million on C-U Hospital, October 10, 1967, University Communications & Public Relations Materials: News Releases. Special Collections & Archives, UC San Diego Library.
7. Dean of UCSD's Medical School to Be Joseph Stokes III, October 18, 1963, University Communications & Public Relations Materials: News Releases. Special Collections & Archives, UC San Diego Library.
8. My Recollections of the Formation of the School of Medicine at UCSD 1961 – 1970, RN Hamburger. Chronicles (Newsletter of the UCSD Emeriti Association), Volume 1, No. 3 (March 2002), pp 3 – 4.
9. Clifford Grobstein Appointment, May 18, 1967, University Communications & Public Relations Materials: News Releases. Special Collections & Archives, UC San Diego Library.

10. Dean Stokes Resigns, September 30, 1966, University Communications & Public Relations Materials: News Releases. Special Collections & Archives, UC San Diego Library.
11. Important Dates and Events in UCSD History (Part of 25th Anniversary Press Kit), October 7, 1985, University Communications & Public Relations Materials: News Releases. Special Collections & Archives, UC San Diego Library.
12. N.K. Wessells: Clifford Grobstein. Biographical Memoirs, Volume 78. National Academy of Sciences. The National Academy of Sciences Press, Washington, D.C., 2000, pp 86-87.
13. Oral History of Robert Hamburger, April 20, 2000, UCSD Oral Histories. Special Collections & Archives, UC San Diego Library.
14. UCSD Medical Students Place First in National Exam, University Bulletin, A Weekly Bulletin for the Staff of the University of California, Volume 20, No. 105, December 13, 1971, p. 64.
15. First Medical Students to Start Classes, September 9, 1968, University Communications & Public Relations Materials: News Releases. Special Collections & Archives, UC San Diego Library.
16. School of Medicine Basic Science Building to Be Dedicated, November 25, 1969, University Communications & Public Relations Materials: News Releases. Special Collections & Archives, UC San Diego Library.
17. Medical School Groundbreaking, September 26, 1966, University Communications & Public Relations Materials: News Releases. Special Collections & Archives, UC San Diego Library.
18. School of Medicine Basic Science Building to Be Dedicated, November 25, 1969, University Communications & Public Relations Materials: News Releases. Special Collections & Archives, UC San Diego Library.
19. Dr. Grobstein to Return to Teaching Position, June 17, 1977, University Communications & Public Relations Materials: News Releases. Special Collections & Archives, UC San Diego Library.
20. Commencement Remarks to the School of Medicine Charter Class, Clifford Grobstein, Ph.D., Dean School of Medicine, June 11, 1972
21. Interview with Dr. Robert Hamburger, October 8, 1984. Interviewer, Dr. Kathryn Ringrose, October 8, 1984, UCSD Oral Histories, Special Collections & Archives, UC San Diego Library.

Chapter 3
Evolution of the Curriculum

The first teaching of the curriculum in this fledgling school was revolutionary, to say the least, establishing the school of medicine as truly thinking "out of the box."

Nearly 30 FTEs (state-funded faculty lines) had been granted to campus departments to teach the basic sciences in the school of medicine [1]. The so-called "participating departments" included Aerospace and Mechanical Engineering Sciences, Biology, Chemistry, Economics, Mathematics, Physics, Psychology, Scripps Institution of Oceanography, and Sociology [2]. Interestingly and perhaps predictably, the "Bonner Plan" started to fall apart with only 21 campus faculty left in the plan by 1980 [3]. This was due in part to waning interest of campus faculty in teaching in the school of medicine coupled with the school of medicine's desire to teach more of the preclinical curriculum itself. In the late 1980's, 6.00 Bonner Plan FTEs were gleaned from the general campus by then UC San Diego Chancellor Richard Atkinson via "buyout" of each occupied FTE by the campus (0.62 FTE went to the school of medicine and 0.38 FTE was retained by the campus) so that many faculty were split between a school of medicine appointment (0.62 FTE) and a "participating department" appointment (0.38 FTE). The 6.00 recovered FTEs were used to strengthen basic science in the school of medicine: 0.5 FTE was given to the Department of Pharmacology, and 5.5 FTEs were given to build a Division of Cellular and Molecular Medicine. The remainder of the FTEs was subsequently returned to the school of medicine either upon retirement of the incumbent faculty member in a "participating" department or the desire of a faculty member to have his/her primary appointment in the school of medicine. These latter FTEs were also used to strengthen basic science in the school of medicine (Department of Pharmacology, Department of Cellular and Molecular Medicine, and selected divisions in the Department of Medicine) [4].

The Inaugural Curriculum

The inaugural curriculum was a "pass-fail" one consisting of five "block" courses (large segments of contiguous time) and three "strip" courses (shorter units offered over the first two years) [Maria Randerson, personal communication and research, March 17, 2017; David N. Bailey, personal recollections and research]:

Year 1

Four block courses: cell biology and biochemistry; basic neurology; organ physiology and pharmacology; and mathematics and physical sciences.

Two strip courses: introduction to clinical medicine (histories, interviewing, physical examination, laboratory examination) and social and behavioral sciences (medical sociology, comparative cultural studies, medical economics, psychological factors).

Electives (about 25% of the time)

Year 2

Two block courses: human anatomy and pathology/microbiology.

Two strip courses: introduction to clinical medicine and social and behavioral sciences.

Electives (about 25% of the time)

Year 3 (Note: at the time of launching the curriculum for the first matriculating students, the clinical disciplines had not yet been offered and were only in the planning stages)

Clinical rotations: surgery, medicine, pediatrics (no others mentioned although a family health program was contemplated as well as summer electives and social and community medicine).

Strip courses: occupational and environmental medicine; disease prevention and control; and public policy.

Electives: none (although students could take electives during the summer following the third year)

Year 4 (Note: in planning at the time of launching the curriculum for the first matriculating students)

Clinical disciplines (one quarter)

Electives (two quarters)

Students were required to select a concentration area to pursue over the first three to four quarters of the curriculum and to have a concentration area committee and preceptor to review progress each quarter. At least two thirds of this elective time was to be spent in courses and experiences relevant to the student's objectives in that area. Students were to complete an "investigative experience" relevant to the concentration area. A report based on original work in the concentration area and written in a format suitable for publication was a requirement. Such reports were submitted to the concentration area committee [Maria Randerson, personal communication and research, March 17, 2017].

Available concentration areas (each with many offerings) included marine and aerospace biomedicine, neuroscience, bioengineering, developmental biology, health systems and administration, microbiology and infectious diseases, and immunobiology and transplantation [Maria Randerson, personal communication and research, March 17, 2017].

The philosophy of the inaugural curriculum was that UC San Diego medical students do not differ from other graduate students. Emphasis was placed on each student's maturity and demonstrated ability for independent study. Students were given broad latitude in course selection based upon their academic performance and career development [Maria Randerson, personal communication and research, March 17, 2017].

Formal examinations were minimized in the curriculum. There were year-end comprehensive examinations tailored to the needs of students within constraints set by licensing boards. Academic standing was determined from these examinations and from evaluations of each student by instructors. Passing the National Board of Medical Examiners examinations was required, but the score did not factor into student standing [Maria Randerson, personal communication and research, March 17, 2017].

The curriculum that evolved was sufficiently rigorous that many of the first graduates of the school said that they felt pressured toward research [3]. In fact, as the curriculum progressed over the years, students spent most of their learning time in the lecture hall (sometimes nearly eight hours per day). Furthermore, in those days there were no learning aids (no podcasts, no note-takers, no online learning aids, minimal educational support services, etc.). Perhaps not surprisingly, the UC San Diego School of Medicine slowly earned the reputation of being the "boot camp" of medical schools with the preclinical curriculum resembling graduate school instead of medical school [David N. Bailey, personal recollections and research].

Program in Medical Education – Health Equity (PRIME – Heq)

After nearly 40 years of essentially the same curriculum, changes began to occur. On August 30, 2007, twelve students enrolled in a new curriculum designed to train physicians interested in caring for the underserved population. The so-called "Program in Medical Education – Health Equity (PRIME-HEq)," launched under the leadership of Sandra Daley, the Assistant Dean for Diversity and Community Partnerships, was one of five UC systemwide medical school programs whose focus was on care of the underserved. Each program was a five-year dual-degree program offering a master's degree in an area of the student's choosing (e.g., business administration, healthcare leadership, clinical research, public health). The UC San Diego program "prepares physicians to provide health services to underserved and at risk populations; increases the number of clinicians, research scientists, and advocates addressing minority health and health disparities; creates a diverse community of scholars that develop, disseminate, and apply new knowledge in minority health and health disparities; and promotes a multidisciplinary community/university partnership to eliminate health disparities and increase health equity" [5, 6]. This program continues to be successful.

Integrated Science Curriculum (ISC)

A revolution in the curriculum occurred three years later (2010) under the leadership of Maria Savoia, Dean for Medical Education, and David Brenner, Vice Chancellor for Health Sciences and Dean of the School of Medicine with the launching of the so-called "Integrated

Science Curriculum" (ISC) [7]. This novel curriculum eliminated more than half of the lecture hours and left the afternoons relatively free for student academic pursuits and clinical activities. More clinical experiences were introduced into the first and second years, and problem- and team-based learning were incorporated. Perhaps, not surprisingly, many faculty objected to the major reduction in lecture hours and in the drastic reduction of course time (e.g., microbiology went from a one-year course integrated with pharmacology and pathology to a five-week course; immunology was allotted 10 days). Pathology, anatomy, histology, and pharmacology were no longer core courses. Instead, they became "threads" woven into the new organ system blocks (courses), each of which had its own director. Thread directors had to coordinate with the respective block directors, each of whom had his/her own view of how the subject should be taught [5].

An important element of the curriculum was the establishment of six academic communities with each incoming student being assigned to one of the communities for the entirety of medical school. Each community was directed by a faculty member, who provided mentoring, counselling, and support. The vertical integration that resulted (four years of students in each community) provided better opportunity for mentoring of students by their more senior peers [7].

Electives still remained as well as the requirement to complete an independent study project, based upon original, independent, and scholarly activity of the student with a written summary provided to the student's committee. In addition, successful completion of steps I and II of the (now renamed) United States Medical Licensing Examination (USMLE) continued as a requirement [7].

The ISC pre-clerkship curriculum occupied six quarters of instruction, spanning the spectrum of health and disease and was primarily organ-focused. Years 1 and 2 encompassed an overarching set of blocks (core courses) comprising "Human Health and Disease," offered in the morning, and "Clinical Foundations" offered in the afternoon [7]:

Year 1

Human Health and Disease: foundations of human biology; cardiovascular I; pulmonary I; gastrointestinal I; renal I; musculoskeletal I; mind, brain, and behavior I; endocrine, reproduction & metabolism I; immunology/hematology; and microbiology.

Clinical Foundations: ambulatory care apprenticeship (longitudinal two-year experience with a clinical preceptor); problem-based learning groups; practice of medicine (physical examination, histories, differential diagnosis).

Year 2

Human Health and Disease: principles of clinical oncology; epidemiology, biostatistics, and medical informatics; arthritis, rheumatic diseases, and dermatology; endocrine, reproduction & metabolism II; cardiovascular II; mind, brain, and behavior II; pulmonary II; renal II; and multi-organ system disorders and integrative cases.

Clinical Foundations (as in Year 1)

Formal instruction in Year 2 was shortened to five quarters in order to provide students with six weeks for comprehensive review and study for the required USMLE step I examination.

Following USMLE step I, students completed one week of "clinical transitions" to prepare them for starting core clinical clerkships.

Year 3

Core clinical clerkships: medicine (12 weeks); surgery (8 weeks); pediatrics (8 weeks); reproductive medicine (6 weeks); psychiatry (6 weeks); neurology (4 weeks); primary care (afternoon per week throughout the year, except during surgery); and clinical selectives (two 2-week selectives, at least one of which was in a surgical specialty or surgery-related field such as surgical pathology).

Year 4

Four quarters of enrollment that includes 12 weeks of direct patient care clerkships (one inpatient, one outpatient, one primary care) and at least 16 weeks of other clinical electives, 2 additional elective months, and completion of the independent study project.

In the winter quarter there was a required "Principles to Practice" course (4 weeks) that revisited basic science principles and their integration into clinical practice.

Grading in the new curriculum was "pass-fail" for pre-clerkship (year 1 and year 2) core courses with no "honors" allowed. For the third-year core clinical clerkships grades were "pass," "fail," "honors," and "near honors." For pre-clerkship (year 1 and year 2) electives grades were "satisfactory" and "unsatisfactory" while for fourth-year clinical electives they were "pass," "fail," and "honors." Selectives (third-year) were graded as "pass-fail" with no "honors" allowed. Finally, in keeping with student desire to deemphasize competition as much as possible, there was no chapter of Alpha Omega Alpha, academic medical honorary, although there was a chapter of the Arnold P. Gold Humanism Society, into which about 15 – 20 third-year medical students were elected each year by their classmates and committed themselves to service projects [6].

Despite concerns of a number of faculty about the radical reform in curriculum, the student performance on the USMLE I examination did not decline and in many years was better than in the original curriculum! Perhaps, most importantly, student satisfaction with the curriculum was overwhelming positive [6]. This curriculum continues successfully today.

Student-Run Free Clinic Project

One of the most transformational additions to the curriculum was the Student-Run Free Clinic Project. In 1996 a small group of UC San Diego medical students and faculty approached a community partner that was working with the homeless and offered to provide some clinical services on a weekly basis. The program, based at the Pacific Beach United Methodist Church, welcomed the project, and clinical services were offered one evening per week after a meal offered by the church. Subsequently a formal affiliation agreement was signed between the University and the church, some supplies and medications were donated, and in January 1997 the Student-Run Free Clinic Project was officially launched [8].

In October 1997 the First Lutheran Church of San Diego offered a second site in downtown San Diego. In October 1998 a third site was opened at Baker Elementary School in Southeast San Diego, and in March 2011 a fourth site was opened at Golden Avenue Elementary School in Lemon Grove. These latter two sites are no longer operational [8].

In addition to clinical care provided by medical students under the supervision of licensed faculty attending physicians, other services were offered: pharmacy, dental, legal, health education, a food program, and acupuncture through affiliations with community partners. In addition to medical students, pharmacy students, predental students, and pre-law students became engaged in clinic activities. All medical students were enrolled in a school of medicine elective ("Community Advocacy") which included didactic and experiential sessions as well as the first five clinic sessions [8].

Medications were provided through both purchase of a limited formulary of medications plus a patient assistance program offered by pharmaceutical companies. There was a formal affiliation agreement between each site and the School of Medicine. Funding was primarily from grants, the UC San Diego Health System, and the School of Medicine. This "safety net for the safety net" became a valued site for individuals training in underserved medicine. Ellen Beck, M.D., Professor of Family Medicine and Public Health, has been the executive director since inception of the clinic [8], which continues to be perhaps the most popular elective in the entire medical school curriculum.

Graduate Programs Sponsored by UC San Diego Health Sciences

The Biomedical Sciences (BMS) Ph.D. program, offering advanced multidisciplinary training in basic and disease-oriented research, was founded in 1970 as the Physiology/Pharmacology Graduate Program since the majority of the faculty were basic and clinical scientists involved in teaching those disciplines for the first-year medical students. Over the years the program expanded to include many additional interests and was renamed the Biomedical Sciences

Program in 1990. It is now an umbrella program with participating faculty in every department of the School of Medicine, as well as the Skaggs School of Pharmacy and Pharmaceutical Sciences, the Division of Biological Sciences, the Moores Cancer Center, the Sanford Burnham Prebys Medical Discovery Institute, the Salk Institute for Biological Studies, the Scripps Research Institute, the La Jolla Institute of Allergy and Immunology, and the Departments of Chemistry/Biochemistry and Bioengineering. The program is the largest of the graduate programs sponsored by Health Sciences, having graduated more than 600 students as of Fall 2016 [9].

The Neurosciences Graduate Program, launched in 1969, has been consistently ranked by the National Research Council of the National Academy of Sciences as one of the top ranking neuroscience graduate programs in the country. It is an interdisciplinary program covering a broad spectrum of subdisciplines in neuroscience and draws faculty from UC San Diego as well as the Salk Institute for Biological Studies, the Scripps Research Institute, and the Sanford Burnham Prebys Medical Discovery Institute [10; Norienne Saign, personal communication, May 8, 2017].

An Experimental Pathology Ph.D. program was established by the Department of Pathology in 1973. The name was changed to Molecular Pathology in 1989 as the program changed direction to focus on the molecular basis of human disease with an appreciation of disease at the levels of pathology and histology. Faculty were drawn from the School of Medicine as well as the Sanford Burnham Prebys Medical Discovery Institute, and the Scripps Research Institute. This program was folded into the Biomedical Sciences Program in 2008 [Norienne Saign, personal communication, May 8, 2017].

Medical Scientist Training Program (MSTP)

The Medical Scientist Training Program (MSTP) graduated its first students in 1972 [11]. National Institutes of Health funding for its training grant began in 1974-1975 [11, 12]. In addition to faculty from UC San Diego the program includes faculty at the Scripps Research Institute, the Salk Institute for Biological Studies, the Sanford Burnham Prebys Medical Discovery Institute, and the La Jolla Institute for Allergy and Immunology. Almost all of the MSTP students are engaged in the Student-Run Free Clinic Project at one time or another, and more than 90% of MSTP graduates have obtained positions as physician-scientists at academic health centers or research institutes [11].

References

1. Oral History of Robert Hamburger, April 20, 2000, UCSD Oral Histories, Special Collection & Archives, UC San Diego Library.
2. UCSD Academic Calendar 1969-1970, Volume 2, Number 3, https://library.ucsd.edu/dc/object/bb1879725x/_1.pdf
3. N.A. Anderson. An Improbable Venture: A History of the University of California, San Diego. The UCSD Press, La Jolla, California, 1993, pp 153-180.
4. D.N. Bailey: Bonner Plan FTE Distribution Document, September 3, 2005.
5. UC San Diego School of Medicine Expands Class Size, Launches New Program in Health Disparities, August 30, 2007, University Communications & Public Relations Materials: News Releases. Special Collections & Archives, UC San Diego Library.
6. UC San Diego School of Medicine Diversity and Community Partnership: Program in Medical Education – Health Equity (PRIME-HEq), https://meded.ucsd.edu/index.cfm/asa/dcp/primeheq/
7. UC San Diego School of Medicine Undergraduate Medical Education, https://meded.ucsd.edu/index.cfm/ugme/curriculum_requirements/core_curriculum/
8. E. Beck: The UCSD Student-Run Free Clinic Project: Transdisciplinary Health Professional Education. Journal of Health Care for the Poor and Underserved 16: 207 – 219 (2005).
9. Biomedical Sciences Graduate Program, http://biomedsci.ucsd.edu/about/
10. Neurosciences, http://apply.grad.ucsd.edu/departments/neurosciences
11. UC San Diego School of Medicine: Medical Scientist Training Program, http://mstp.ucsd.edu/welcome/pages/default.aspx

12. MSTP Study: The Careers and Professional Activities of Graduates of the NIGMS Medical Scientist Training Program. Publications.nigms.nih.gov. 2011-04-22.

Chapter 4

Shakers and Movers: The Founding Faculty

(1964 – 1969)

In 1964, Dean Stokes began the recruitment of faculty to the new school of medicine. At that time he was the only faculty member!   He realized that, before recruiting the founding department chairs, he needed an ally to help.

Stokes turned to Robert N. Hamburger, M.D., who was visiting associate professor of biology (visiting from the University of Rochester), as the assistant dean of the school of medicine. Dr. Hamburger had received his Doctor of Medicine degree from Yale and was a board-certified pediatrician. His area of specialty was pediatric allergy and immunology. His charge was to work on planning and development of the school of medicine [David N. Bailey, personal recollections and research; 1].   At that time Stokes and Hamburger were the only faculty members in the school of medicine [2]!

The Founding Department Chairs

The original departments in the school of medicine were nine in number: medicine, neurosciences, obstetrics & gynecology, pathology, pediatrics, preventive medicine, psychiatry, radiology, and surgery. The founding chairs were an illustrious group indeed!

The first department chair to be recruited was Robert Livingston, M.D. in July 1965 as the founding chair of the Department of Neurosciences. This new department would integrate neurobiology, neuroanatomy, neurophysiology, neuropathology, and clinical neurology. Livingston had received both his Doctor of Medicine degree and his residency training at

Stanford University. When recruited to UC San Diego, he was Chief of the General Diseases Research Support Branch of the Division of Research Facilities and Resources and was also Associate Division Chief for Program Planning at the National Institutes of Health. His research focus was brain-mapping [David N. Bailey, personal recollections and research; 2].

Later in 1965 Marshall J. Orloff, M.D. was appointed founding chair of the Department of Surgery at age 38. He was a Markle Scholar in Academic Medicine at UC Los Angeles and professor and chief of surgery at Harbor General Hospital in Los Angeles. A general surgeon, he had received his Doctor of Medicine degree from the University of Illinois at Chicago and had completed his surgery residency at the University of Pennsylvania. At the time of his appointment the school had planned that the department would teach anatomy, a commitment which continues to this day [3]. Orloff espoused the strict full-time salary plan (i.e., faculty being paid according to academic rank and step instead of by practice income). As part of his recruitment package a surgery research building was constructed on the Hillcrest campus [David N. Bailey, personal recollections and research; 4].

As was noted in chapter 2, Joseph Stokes, M.D., became the founding chair of the Department of Preventive Medicine (forerunner of Community and Family Medicine) when he stepped down as founding dean in 1966. His research interests were in preventive medicine and cardiovascular epidemiology [David N. Bailey, personal recollections and research]. As dean he had been responsible for recruiting chairs Livingston and Orloff. The subsequent founding chairs noted below were recruited by Dean Grobstein.

In 1967 Averill Liebow, M.D. was recruited from the Yale faculty to be the founding chair of the Department of Pathology. As the story goes, Robert Hamburger went back to his *alma mater* Yale to seek advice on whom to recruit as chair of pathology. When he asked Averill Liebow, Dr. Liebow offered himself [4]. Liebow was a "true-blue Yalie," having received his Doctor of Medicine degree and his residency training in Pathology at Yale and was an internationally recognized pulmonary pathologist. He was a colorful person known for his strict views of teaching and administration. When faculty would ask to be excused from teaching in order to present an abstract at a national meeting, they were told that their first duty was teaching and that they would have to miss the meeting. It was also rumored that he would perform weekend "rounds" of the parking lot to see which of his faculty were at work (he had memorized the makes of their cars and had a list of their license plate numbers) [Henry C. Powell, personal communication, May 9, 2017]. Dr. Liebow remained chair until a stroke that occurred while he was lecturing to medical students in 1975 incapacitated him. Reportedly he began speaking in German as the stroke occurred [David N. Bailey, personal recollections and research].

In 1968 Eugene Braunwald, M.D. was recruited to be the inaugural chair of the Department of Medicine. A noted research cardiologist, Braunwald had received his Doctor of Medicine degree from New York University and had completed his residency in medicine at Mount Sinai and Johns Hopkins medical centers.   When recruited to UC San Diego he was a clinical director at the National Heart Institute and clinical professor of medicine at Georgetown University [David N. Bailey, personal recollections and research; 6].

In the same year (1968) Elliott Lasser, M.D. became founding chair of the Department of Radiology. He had received his Doctor of Medicine degree from the University of Buffalo and had completed his residency in radiology at the University of Minnesota. His areas of expertise were neuroradiology and gastrointestinal radiology. Prior to his arrival at UC San Diego Dr. Lasser was chair of the Department of Radiology at the University of Pittsburgh [David N. Bailey, personal recollections and research; 7].

Interestingly, and not known by many, Robert Hamburger himself served as founding chair of the Department of Pediatrics for the year 1968-69. In 1969 William Nyhan, M.D., Ph.D. was recruited as the permanent chair of the department. An internationally recognized biochemical geneticist known from his early discovery of the defect causing Lesch-Nyhan syndrome, Nyhan had received his Doctor of Medicine degree from Columbia University College of Physicians and Surgeons and his Doctor of Philosophy degree from the University of Illinois. He completed his residency in pediatrics at Yale University. At the time of his appointment as chair at UC San Diego, Dr. Nyhan was chair of the Department of Pediatrics at the University of Miami [8].

In 1969 Arnold Mandell, M.D. was appointed founding chair of the Department of Psychiatry. He had received his Doctor of Medicine degree at Tulane University and had completed a residency at UC Los Angeles Neuropsychiatric Institute. When he was attracted from the UC Irvine faculty to become chair at UC San Diego he was purportedly the youngest physician ever appointed as chair of a department of psychiatry (age 35). Under Dr. Mandell's leadership the department became the first department of psychiatry to become biologically oriented [9].

The last of the founding chairs to be recruited was Kenneth Ryan, M.D., who became chair of

the Department of Obstetrics & Gynecology (later to be renamed Reproductive Medicine) in

1970. He had received his Doctor of Medicine degree from Harvard and had completed an

internal medicine residency at both Massachusetts General Hospital and Columbia-Presbyterian

Hospitals followed by a residency in obstetrics and gynecology at the Boston Lying-In Hospital

and Free Hospital for Women. At the time of his recruitment to UC San Diego Dr. Ryan was

chair of the Department of Obstetrics and Gynecology at Case Western Reserve University. His

research focused on the biology of steroidogenesis. He was the shortest serving of the

founding UC San Diego School of Medicine chairs, leaving in 1972 to return to Harvard as chair

of Obstetrics, Gynecology, and Reproductive Biology [David N. Bailey, personal recollections

and research; 10].

Other Founding Faculty

With the founding department chairs in place, the recruitment of the early founding faculty

began in earnest. In the period following the appointment of Robert Hamburger in 1964 (see

above) through 1969, many other distinguished founding faculty were recruited to UC San

Diego. Then, starting in 1970, a veritable "tidal wave" of new faculty, both senior and junior

would start to be lured to UC San Diego.

In addition to the department chairs and deans previously mentioned, the following

founding faculty were recruited to UC San Diego School of Medicine by 1970 (arranged

alphabetically by last name): Wayne Akeson, M.D. (Professor of Surgery/Orthopedics),

Toshiyuki Ando, M.D. (Assistant Professor of Pediatrics), William Ashburn, M.D. (Assistant

Professor of Radiology/Nuclear Medicine), Norman Baily, Ph.D. (Professor of

Radiology/Radiation Physics), Samuel Barondes, M.D. (Professor of Psychiatry), Elizabeth

Barrett-Connor, M.D. (Assistant Professor of Medicine), Henrik Bendixen, M.D. (Professor of

Surgery/Anesthesiology), Kurt Benirschke, M.D. (Professor of Obstetrics and Gynecology and

Pathology), Eugene Bernstein, M.D., Ph.D. (Professor of Surgery/Cardiothoracic Surgery),

Reginald Bickford, M.D. (Professor of Neurosciences/Neurophysiology), Colin M. Bloor, M.D.

(Assistant Professor of Pathology/Cardiac Pathology), Abraham Braude, M.D. (Professor of

Medicine/Infectious Diseases), Nina Braunwald, M.D. (Associate Professor of

Surgery/Cardiothoracic Surgery), Charles Bridgeman, Ph.D. (Assistant Professor of

Neurosciences/Anatomy and Learning Resources), Kenneth Brown, M.D. (Assistant Professor of

Medicine), Virgil Brown, M.D. (Assistant Professor of Medicine), Theodore Bullock, Ph.D.

(Professor of Neurosciences/Neurophysiology), Charles Carrington, M.D. (Assistant Professor of

Pathology/Pulmonary Pathology), James Connor, M.D. (Associate Professor of Pediatrics),

James Covell, M.D. (Assistant Professor of Medicine/Cardiology), John Davis, M.D. (Assistant

Professor of Obstetrics and Gynecology), Ralph Dilley, M.D. (Assistant Professor of Surgery), J.L.

Doppman (Professor of Radiology/Interventional Radiology), Max Elliott, M.D. (Assistant

Professor of Pathology), Darrell Fanestil, M.D. (Associate Professor of Medicine/Nephrology),

Paul Friedman, M.D. (Assistant Professor of Radiology/Thoracic Radiology), William Friedman,

M.D. (Assistant Professor of Pediatrics/Cardiology), Theodore Friedmann, M.D. (Assistant

Professor of Pediatrics), Robert Galambos, M.D., Ph.D. (Professor of

Neurosciences/Neuroelectrophysiology), Leonard Garren (Professor of

Medicine/Endocrinology), James Gault, M.D. (Assistant Professor of Medicine), Samuel

Giammona, M.D. (Professor of Pediatrics/Pulmonology), Gordon Gill, M.D. (Assistant Professor of Medicine/Endocrinology and Metabolism), Ruben Gittes, M.D. (Associate Professor of Surgery/Urology), Louis Gluck, M.D. (Professor of Pediatrics/Neonatology), Mehran Goulian, M.D. (Professor of Medicine/Hematology), Richard Gross, M.D. (Assistant Professor of Medicine), James Hagadorn, M.D. (Assistant Professor of Medicine in Residence), Nicholas Halasz, M.D. (Associate Professor of Surgery/Anatomy), Cecil Hougie, M.D. (Professor of Pathology/Hemostasis), Peter Hutchin, M.D. (Assistant Professor of Surgery), Harvey Itano, M.D., Ph.D. (Professor of Pathology), Oliver W. Jones, M.D. (Associate Professor of Medicine/Cytogenetics), Lewis Judd, M.D. (Associate Professor of Psychiatry), Marvin Karno, M.D. (Assistant Professor of Psychiatry), Arnold Kisch, M.D. (Associate Professor of Community Medicine), Alexis Kniazeff, D.V.M., Ph.D. (Professor of Medicine), Faith Kung, M.D. (Assistant Professor of Pediatrics in Residence), Peter W. Lampert, M.D. (Professor of Pathology/Neuropathology), G. David Lange, Ph.D. (Assistant Professor of Neurosciences), Sun Lee, M.D. (Associate Professor of Surgery in Residence), Allen Lein, Ph.D. (Professor of Reproductive Medicine/Endocrinology), Richard Mani, M.D. (Assistant Professor of Radiology), Serafeim Masouredis, M.D., Ph.D. (Professor of Pathology/Transfusion Medicine), Steven Mayer, Ph.D. (Professor of Medicine/Pharmacology), John Mendelsohn, M.D. (Assistant Professor of Medicine), Katsumi Miyai, M.D., Ph.D. (Assistant Professor of Pathology/Gastrointestinal Pathology), Kenneth Moser, M.D. (Associate Professor of Medicine/Pulmonology), James Nelson, M.D. (Associate Professor of Neurosciences), John O'Brien, M.D. (Associate Professor of Neurosciences), Robert O'Rourke, M.D. (Assistant Professor of Medicine), Stanley Pappelbaum, M.D. (Assistant Professor of Medicine and

Pediatrics), Nolan Penn, M.D. (Professor of Psychiatry), Richard Peters, M.D. (Professor of

Surgery/Cardiothoracic Surgery), Peter Pool, M.D. (Assistant Professor of Medicine), Stewart

Reuter, M.D. (Associate Professor of Radiology), Roger Rosenberg, M.D. (Assistant Professor of

Neurosciences), John Ross, Jr., M.D. (Professor of Medicine/Cardiology), James Schauble, M.D.

(Associate Professor of Surgery), Jerry Schneider, M.D. (Assistant Professor of Pediatrics),

Lawrence Schneiderman, M.D. (Associate Professor of Community Medicine and Medicine), J.

Edwin Seegmiller, M.D. (Professor of Medicine/Metabolism), Stewart Sell, M.D. (Associate

Professor of Pathology), Michael Shimkin, M.D. (Professor of Community Medicine), Allan

Simon, M.D. (Associate Professor of Radiology), Harold Simon, M.D., Ph.D. (Assistant Professor

of Community Medicine), Burton Sobel (Assistant Professor of Medicine/Cardiology), Charles

Spooner, Ph.D. (Assistant Professor of Neurosciences), Daniel Steinberg, M.D. Ph.D. (Professor

of Medicine/Endocrinology and Metabolism), Harley Sybers, M.D. (Assistant Professor of

Pathology), Lee Talner, M.D. (Assistant Professor of Radiology/Diagnostic Radiology), John

Thorson, M.D. (Assistant Professor of Neurosciences), Gennaro Tisi, M.D. (Assistant Professor of

Medicine/Pulmonology), Robert Tschirgi, M.D., Ph.D. (Professor of Neurosciences), Carl

vonEssen, M.D. (Professor of Radiology/Radiotherapy), John West, M.D. (Professor of

Medicine/Pulmonology), Henry Wheeler, M.D. (Professor of Medicine/Gastroenterology),

Sanford Wolf, M.D. (Assistant Professor of Psychiatry), Samuel Yen, M.D. (Professor of

Obstetrics and Gynecology), Richard Yoder, M.D. (Assistant Professor of Community Medicine),

Charles York, D.V.M., Ph.D. (Associate Professor of Pathology), Alfred Zettner, M.D. (Professor

of Pathology/Clinical Pathology), and Nathan Zvaifler, M.D. (Professor of Medicine) [David N.

Bailey, personal recollections and research; 11 – 14].

Complementing these founding faculty were the following 32 "Bonner Plan" faculty in the

"participating departments": William Allison, Ph.D. (Assistant Professor of Chemistry), Alan

Bearden, Ph.D. (Assistant Professor of Chemistry), Alan Cicourel, Ph.D. (Professor of Sociology),

Edward Dennis, Ph.D. (Assistant Professor of Chemistry), J. Anthony Deutsch, Ph.D. (Professor

of Psychology), Russell Doolittle, Ph.D. (Assistant Professor of Chemistry), Richard Dutton,

Ph.D. (Associate Professor of Biology), John Elovson, Ph.D. (Assistant Professor of Biology), John

Evans, Ph.D. (Assistant Professor of Mathematics), Edmund Fantino, Ph.D. (Assistant Professor

of Psychology), Morris Friedkin, Ph.D. (Professor of Biology), Arnost Fronek, M.D., Ph.D.

(Associate Professor of Aerospace and Mechanical Engineering Sciences), Yuan-Chen Fung,

Ph.D. (Professor of Aerospace and Mechanical Engineering Sciences), Adriano Garsia, Ph.D.

(Professor of Mathematics), Peter Geiduschek, Ph.D. (Professor of Biology),   Ronald Getoor,

Ph.D. (Professor of Mathematics), Clifford Grobstein, Ph.D. (Dean; Professor of Biology),

Susumu Hagiwara, M.D., Ph.D. (Professor, Scripps Institution of Oceanography), Harold

Hammel, Ph.D. (Professor, Scripps Institution of Oceanography), Seymour Harris, Ph.D.

(Professor of Economics), Marcos Intaglietta, Ph.D. (Assistant Professor of Aerospace and

Mechanical Engineering Sciences), Nathan Kaplan, Ph.D. (Professor of Chemistry), Dan Lindsley,

Ph.D. (Professor of Biology), William McGuire, Ph.D. (Professor of Psychology), Xuong Nguyen-

Huu, Ph.D. (Assistant Professor of Physics and Biology), Thomas O'Neil, Ph.D. (Assistant

Professor of Physics), Paul Price, Ph.D. (Assistant Professor of Biology), Arthur Robinson, Ph.D.

(Assistant Professor of Biology), Thomas Roth, Ph.D. (Assistant Professor of Biology), Percy

Russell, Ph.D. (Associate Professor of Biology), Silvio Varon, M.D., Eng.D. (Associate Professor of

Biology), and Benjamin Zweifach, Ph.D. (Professor of Aerospace and Mechanical Engineering

Sciences) [11 – 14].

First School of Medicine Administrators

In addition to these founding chairs and faculty, before the end of his term as Dean, Clifford

Grobstein had assembled a strong team of faculty administrators to guide the fledgling school:

associate dean for administration (Allen Lein, Ph.D.), assistant dean for curriculum and faculty

affairs (Robert N. Hamburger, M.D.), assistant dean for student affairs (Harold Simon, M.D.,

Ph.D.), program director for basic sciences in medicine (Daniel Steinberg, M.D., Ph.D.), director

and assistant dean for learning resources (Charles Bridgeman, Ph.D.), and director of the

division of animal resources (Charles York, D.V.M., Ph.D.) [Maria Randerson, personal

communication, March 17, 2017].

References

1. Appointments of Dr. R.N. Hamburger and Dr. S.J. Singer, May 13, 1964. In "News Releases," Series Two of the University Communications & Public Relations Materials. RSS 6020. Special Collections & Archives, UC San Diego Library.
2. Livingston & Lockwood Join School of Medicine Staff, June 24, 1965, , University Communications & Public Relations Materials: News Releases. Special Collections & Archives, UC San Diego Library.
3. Dr. Marshall J. Orloff Accepts Chairmanship of Department of Surgery at School of Medicine at University of California, San Diego, November 15, 1965, University Communications & Public Relations Materials: News Releases. Special Collections & Archives, UC San Diego Library.
4. Oral History of Robert Hamburger, April 20, 2000, UCSD Oral Histories. Special Collection & Archives, UC San Diego Library.
5. USCAP, About Past Presidents: Averill A. Liebow, 1953-54, https://www.uscap.org/about/history/past-presidents/averill-a-liebow
6. Dr. Eugene Braunwald is PILS lecturer, January 31, 1969. University Communications & Public Relations Materials: News Releases. Special Collections & Archives, UC San Diego Library.

7. Dr. Elliott C. Lasser Appointed As Professor and Chairman of the Department of Radiology at UCSD School of Medicine, June 18, 1968, University Communications & Public Relations Materials: News Releases. Special Collections & Archives, UC San Diego Library.

8. Pediatric History Center, American Academy of Pediatrics, Oral History Project: William L. Nyhan, M.D., Ph.D., Interviewed by Laurence Finberg, M.D., March 3, 2004. American Academy of Pediatrics, Elk Grove Village, Illinois, 2011.

9. Arnold J. Mandell: Interview by David Healy, December 13, 1998, https://www.google.com/?gws_rd=ssl#q=arnold+mandell+interview+david+healy&spf=78

10. Physicians for Reproductive Health: Kenneth J. Ryan, M.D., https://prh.org/provider-voices/kenneth-j-ryan-md-memorial-program/programs-kenneth-j-ryan-md/

11. UCSD Academic Calendar 1967-1968.

12. UCSD Academic Calendar 1968-1969, Volume 1, Number 1.

13. UCSD Academic Calendar 1969-1970, Volume 2, Number 3.

14. UCSD Academic Calendar 1970-1971, Volume 3, Number 2.

Chapter 5

Fifty Years of Deans and Department Chairs
(1967 – 2018)

Following the resignation of Joseph Stokes as dean of the school of medicine in 1966 the next fifty years saw the school's rapid rise to prominence under a series of outstanding deans and department chairs. This chapter will track that progress except for construction of buildings. Clinical buildings will be included in chapter 6, and research and educational buildings will be discussed in chapter 7.

Clifford Grobstein (1967 – 1973)

During the final years of Clifford Grobstein's tenure as dean several department chair changes occurred as founding chairs left. In 1970 John O'Brien, M.D., UC San Diego professor of neurosciences and a distinguished basic neuroscientist known for his discovery of the genetic basis of Tay Sachs disease and development of a screening test for the disease [1], replaced Robert Livingston, M.D. as chair of the Department of Neurosciences when the latter stepped down to return to the faculty [1].

The year 1972 saw the "raiding" of two department chairs by Harvard. Eugene Braunwald, M.D. left as chair of the Department of Medicine to become chair of the Department of Medicine and Chief of Medicine at Brigham & Women's Hospital. Dean Grobstein then appointed Nathan ("Nate") Zvaifler, M.D., head of the UC San Diego Division of Rheumatology, as interim chair of medicine (1972-73) [2, 3]. Also, in 1972, Samuel Yen, M.D., Sc.D., world-renowned reproductive endocrinologist, replaced Kenneth Ryan, M.D. as chair of the

Department of Reproductive Medicine. Dr. Ryan left after only two years as chair in order to become chair of the Department of Obstetrics, Gynecology, and Reproductive Biology at Harvard [4]. Trained at both Johns Hopkins and Harvard, Dr. Yen was a professor at Case Western Reserve University prior to his recruitment to UC San Diego [5].

John Moxley (1973 – 1979)

Following the resignation of Clifford Grobstein as vice chancellor for medicine and biological sciences and dean of the school of medicine, John ("Jack") Moxley III, M.D. was appointed Vice Chancellor for Health Sciences and Dean of the School of Medicine. Moxley had been dean of the University of Maryland School of Medicine for four years, at that time being the youngest dean (age 34) in the United States [6]. He brought with him V. Wayne Kennedy as assistant vice chancellor for health sciences and Margaret Jackson as assistant to the dean [7].

Under Moxley's leadership the school of medicine secured nearly $30 million to expand the school of medicine and the medical center, and he oversaw the opening of the Clinical Teaching Facility (actually mostly research laboratories) in Hillcrest and the Medical Teaching Facility (mostly research laboratories and school of medicine administration) in La Jolla. Moxley also spearheaded the development of the Gildred Cancer Center in Hillcrest and its establishment as a National Institutes of Health designated specialized cancer center. He also helped to obtain a 10-year maximum accreditation of the school of medicine by the Liaison Committee on Medical Education. In addition he initiated discussions with Children's Hospital of San Diego about a formal affiliation between the two institutions, and on his watch the "University Hospital of San Diego County" was renamed the "University of California Medical Center" [6].

During Moxley's deanship Anesthesiology, a division headed by Henrik Bendixen in the Department of Surgery, was split out and became a department in 1974 with Lawrence Saidman, M.D., professor on the anesthesiology service at University Hospital, as founding chair [Gerard Manecke, personal communication, February 14, 2017]. Then a series of chair recruitments kept Moxley quite busy.

Helen M. Ranney, M.D. was appointed chair of the Department of Medicine in 1973 [2]. Dr. Ranney, elected to the National Academy of Sciences that same year, was an internationally recognized hematologist who was the first woman to chair an academic department of medicine in the United States and the first to describe the abnormal blood-cell structure and genetic factors associated with sickle cell disease. She subsequently would also become the first woman Distinguished Physician of the Veterans Administration. She had been professor at the State University of New York at Buffalo when she was recruited to UC San Diego [8]. Doris Howell, M.D., chair of the Department of Pediatrics at the Medical College of Pennsylvania and a noted pediatric hematologist, replaced founding chair Joseph Stokes as Chair in the newly renamed Department of Community and Family Medicine in 1974 [9]. Following the stroke of founding chair Averill Liebow in 1975, Colin Bloor, M.D., UC San Diego professor of pathology, served as interim chair of the Department of Pathology (1975 – 1977) until Kurt Benirschke, M.D., professor of pathology, was appointed (some say "coerced" into being) chair in 1977 [10]. Benirschke had been chair of the Department of Pathology at Dartmouth for ten years, assuming that role at age 35, before he stepped down and joined the UC San Diego faculty as a professor of pathology in 1970 in order to pursue his research in reproductive endocrinology and to help found the Department of Reproductive Medicine (then known as Obstetrics and

Gynecology) [David N. Bailey, personal recollections and research]. Also in 1977 Lewis Judd, M.D., UC San Diego professor of psychiatry, succeeded founding chair Arnold Mandell, M.D. as chair of the Department of Psychiatry and was destined to be the longest serving chair in the school (36 years) [11] while Robert Berk, M.D., Chair of Radiology at the University of Texas, Southwestern, was appointed UC San Diego chair in the same year, succeeding founding chair Elliott Lasser [12]. In 1978 John O'Brien stepped down as chair of the Department of Neurosciences, and Wigbert ("Bert") Wiederholt, M.D., UC San Diego professor of neurosciences, replaced him, being the first clinician to serve in that capacity [David N. Bailey, personal recollections and research]. Finally, in 1979, Peter W. Lampert, M.D., UC San Diego professor of pathology and head of the Division of Neuropathology, was appointed chair of the Department of Pathology following Kurt Benirschke's resignation after only two years as chair [David N. Bailey, personal recollections and research].

After a busy period of recruiting chairs, Dean Moxley took a a one-year leave of absence in the office of the Assistant Secretary of Defense for Health Affairs. Then in 1979 he resigned as vice chancellor and dean to assume the post of Assistant Secretary of Defense for Health Affairs, an appointment made by President Jimmy Carter [6]. Interestingly, Moxley's departure followed quickly upon the heels of the resignation of Chancellor McElroy, in whom a vote of "no confidence" had been rendered by the Academic Senate (allegedly due to McElroy's support of Moxley's attempt to force the resignation of surgery department chair Marshall Orloff over control of the department's not-for-profit Surgery and Education Research Fund that covered expenses for faculty such as travel) [13].

Marvin Dunn (1979 – 1980) and William Hollingsworth (1980 – 1981)

With the departure of Dean Moxley, Marvin Dunn, M.D., associate dean for academic affairs in the school of medicine, was appointed interim vice chancellor and dean. During that year discussions involving the purchase of the medical center from the County of San Diego were launched. However, Dunn's service was cut short when he was appointed dean of the school of medicine at the University of Texas, San Antonio [David N. Bailey, personal recollections and research; 14, 15]. Accordingly, newly appointed Chancellor Richard Atkinson (who had been recruited from the National Science Foundation, where he was director) appointed William Hollingsworth, M.D., Chief of Medicine at the Veterans Affairs San Diego Healthcare System, as interim vice chancellor and dean [David N. Bailey, personal recollections and research; 15] while the search for a permanent vice chancellor and dean continued. In 1981 Dr. Hollingsworth appointed Elizabeth Barrett-Connor, M.D., professor and head of the Division of Epidemiology, to be the interim chair of the Department of Community and Family Medicine when Doris Howell stepped down to return to the faculty [David N. Bailey, personal recollections and research].

Robert G. Petersdorf (1981 – 1986)

After a rather protracted search, Chancellor Atkinson appointed Robert G. Petersdorf, M.D. as vice chancellor and dean. Petersdorf was a legend in American medicine. He had received his Doctor of Medicine degree at Yale in 1952 and had completed residency training in internal medicine at Yale and Harvard as well as subsequent training in infectious diseases at Johns Hopkins. During his chief residency at Yale he began working on a paper describing 100 patients who had been ill for more than three weeks and who had episodic fever of more than 101 degrees. Published with his mentor, Paul Beeson, chair of the Department of Medicine at Yale, this 1961 classic paper [16] described "fever of unexplained origin" and is one of the most frequently cited papers in the medical literature. About the same time Petersdorf assumed his first faculty position as the first and only full-time faculty member at what is now Harborview Medical Center affiliated with the University of Washington. Four years later he became the second chair of the Department of Medicine at the University of Washington at the age of 38, one of the youngest chairs in the nation. During his 15-year tenure as chair (1964 – 1979) he expanded the number of faculty from 69 to 322 full-time faculty. In 1968 he also assumed the editorship of Harrison's Principles of Internal Medicine, holding that position for 22 years. Just prior to coming to UC San Diego (1979 - 1981) Dr. Petersdorf was president of Brigham & Women's Hospital and professor of medicine at Harvard [17].

Except for Joseph Stokes all previous deans had also had the title of vice chancellor for health sciences. However, they had not had authority over the medical center, whose director had reported directly to the chancellor of UC San Diego. That changed with Petersdorf's arrival when he recruited Robert Erra in 1982 to be the director of UC San Diego Medical Center, reporting directly to him for most matters, with Chancellor Atkinson's approval of course [David N. Bailey, personal recollections and research].

Petersdorf's reputation as a tough administrator and change-agent preceded him, much to the fear of the department chairs. In fact, Peter W. Lampert, chair of pathology, suggested that the chairs submit their resignations *en masse* in order to permit Petersdorf free reign to retain the chairs he wanted or to recruit new ones. Needless to say, no chairs actually followed through on that proposal [David N. Bailey, personal recollections and research]. That said, Petersdorf did recruit a number of new chairs and appointed some interim chairs during his term as vice chancellor and dean.

In 1982 Dean Petersdorf appointed interim chair Elizabeth Barrett-Connor, M.D. to be permanent chair of the Department of Community and Family Medicine [David N. Bailey, personal recollections and research]. In 1983 Petersdorf recruited Stuart Brown, M.D., professor and chair of the Department of Ophthalmology at the University of Pittsburgh, to be chair of the newly created Department of Ophthalmology, which had previously been a division in the Department of Surgery [David N. Bailey, personal recollections and research]. That same year (1983) he appointed Robert Resnick, M.D., professor and Head of the Division of Obstetrics since 1974, to be chair of the Department of Reproductive Medicine, succeeding Samuel Yen when he returned to the faculty [David N. Bailey, personal recollections and research; Charles Nager, personal communication, February 15, 2017]. Rounding out a "triple-hitter year" of recruitment, in 1983 Petersdorf appointed A.R. Moossa, M.D., professor and head of the Division of General Surgery at the University of Chicago, to chair the Department of Surgery after Marshall Orloff decided that it was time to step down as chair. Affectionately known as "Babs" by his colleagues, Dr. Moossa was well known for his chain-smoking of cigars and his many colorful quips (the so-called "Moossa's rules") which were numbered and recounted to trainees and others on almost a daily basis. One, recalled by the author, was: "there are only 24 hours in a day, and, if you can't get your work done in that time, you must work overtime!" [David N. Bailey, personal recollections and research]. Finally, in 1983 Dr. Petersdorf appointed Doris Trauner, M.D., professor and head of the Division of Pediatric Neurology, as interim chair of the Department of Neurosciences following the death of Wigbert Wiederholt from cancer [David N. Bailey, personal recollections and research]. In 1984, he recruited Robert Katzman, M.D., chair of the Department of Neurology at the Albert Einstein College of Medicine, to be the permanent chair of the Department of Neurosciences. Katzman was instrumental in establishing one of the five original Alzheimer's Disease Research Centers through National Institute on Aging funding [David N. Bailey, personal recollections and research; 18].

In 1985 Petersdorf appointed George Leopold, M.D., professor of radiology and a nationally renowned pioneer in ultrasonography, as chair of the Department of Radiology, succeeding Robert Berk, M.D. who had resigned as chair [David N. Bailey, personal recollections and research]. In 1986 he appointed Harvey Shapiro, M.D., professor of anesthesiology and expert in neuro-anesthesiology, as chair of the Department of Anesthesiology to follow Lawrence Saidman, when the latter stepped down to join the faculty at Stanford [Gerard Manecke, personal communication, February 14, 2017]. A little later in the same year Petersdorf appointed Michael Kaback, M.D., professor and medical geneticist at the Harbor-UC Los Angeles Medical Center, to succeed William Nyhan, when the latter returned to the faculty. Dr. Kaback had collaborated with John O'Brien during the latter's sabbatical leave at Johns Hopkins, and he shared O'Brien's interest in Tay-Sachs disease [David N. Bailey, personal recollections and research; Gabriel Haddad, personal communication, February 15, 2017; 19].

Also, in 1986, Petersdorf appointed two interim chairs: Stephen Wasserman, M.D., professor and Head of the Division of Allergy, to succeed Helen Ranney, with whom Petersdorf had a rather tense relationship, as Chair of the Department of Medicine, when she became the first women Distinguished Physician in the Veterans Affairs Healthcare System [9]; and David N. Bailey, M.D., Professor of Pathology, Head of the Division of Laboratory Medicine, and Director of Clinical Laboratories, to succeed Peter W. Lampert as interim chair of the Department of Pathology when the latter succumbed to cancer [David N. Bailey, personal recollections and research].

Perhaps one of Petersdorf's most significant accomplishments was to set the stage for establishment of the first basic science department in the school (pharmacology, which was a division in the Department of Medicine at the time). This was stimulated in part by concern that other universities were becoming interested in the division director, Palmer Taylor, Ph.D. and what his talents might offer them. Despite that, some Department of Medicine faculty voiced concerns that this action might start a trend of basic-science divisions breaking away from the clinical departments in which they were embedded, thereby losing synergy with the clinical divisions of the department. With the strong support of department chair Ranney and after going through due process to create a department, departmental status was granted to Pharmacology with Palmer Taylor, Ph.D. as the founding chair. While the groundwork for departmental status was laid in 1986, Palmer Taylor did not assume the chair until 1987 [David N. Bailey, personal recollections and research; Palmer W. Taylor, personal communication, May 22, 2017].

Petersdorf, affectionately known as "the Dorf" by many, was a self-proclaimed insomniac who often had a very tired, worn-looking mien. He found solace in swimming daily at lunchtime, then returning to the office for the continuation of his unusually long days. To the many people who reported to him, including yours truly, Petersdorf was an austere and daunting individual on the outside but a warm-hearted, caring person on the inside [David N. Bailey, personal recollections and research]. A vivid recollection is when the author, then director of clinical laboratories and prior to having been appointed interim chair of pathology, was trying to straighten out thorny issues regarding other school of medicine departmentally based clinical laboratory operations (some 32 in number) that were not appropriately licensed to operate in the State of California. Knowing that this could be an uphill battle especially since some of the illegally operating laboratories were run by department chairs, the author met with Dr. Petersdorf to ask his backing for making those laboratories compliant with the state law. Petersdorf reponded by lowering his glasses and saying: "My son, at Harvard we had many such laboratories and they actually were quite good." Garnering my courage I replied: "With all due respect, Dr. Petersdorf, this is not Harvard, and it is not Massachusetts. This is California." With that, Petersdorf said: "Okay, I support you. You have my backing" [David N. Bailey, personal recollections and research].

Petersdorf's persuasive manner was exemplified by yet another anecdote. In a meeting with the department chairs, a lively debate was conducted about where to place the long-discussed campus hospital. A majority of the chairs wanted it to be located on the west campus so that faculty could leave their academic offices and laboratories and quickly arrive at the hospital. Being the visionary that he was, Petersdorf held out for the then, almost completely vacant, east campus, indicating that there would be not be sufficient room for growth of the clinical enterprise on the west campus and that there would not be room for much further growth of basic science on the west campus if the hospital were located there. That reasoning satisfied both the more clinically oriented chairs and the more basic-science oriented chairs, with the chairs agreeing that the campus hospital would be located on the east campus [David N. Bailey, personal recollections and research].

In late summer of 1986, Dr. Petersdorf announced his departure to become President of the Association of American Medical Colleges (AAMC) [13]. In this role he would make a major impact in American medicine by advocating that medical schools should limit the number of specialists they trained and should focus on training primary care physicians. He also focused on increasing diversity in the medical school student body and faculty. In 1995 he returned to the faculty of the University of Washington and also served as Distinguished Physician at the Veterans Affairs Puget Sound Healthcare System [20].

Wayne Akeson (1986 – 1988)

On the departure of Robert Petersdorf, Chancellor Atkinson appointed Wayne Akeson, M.D., professor and head of the Division of Orthopaedic Surgery, as interim vice chancellor and dean during another protracted search for a permanent vice chancellor and dean [21].

Gerard N. Burrow (1988 – 1992)

After a national search Chancellor Atkinson appointed Gerard N. Burrow, M.D., chair of the Department of Medicine at the University of Toronto and physician-in-chief of Toronto General Hospital, as the vice chancellor and dean. A noted thyroid endocrinologist, Burrow was instrumental in expanding the clinical practice and in developing and opening the long-awaited campus hospital in 1993 (the John M and Sally B Thornton Hospital to be described later) [22]. Among Dean Burrow's additional accomplishments was the creation of a series of "deans" for functional areas: clinical affairs (Harvey Shapiro, M.D., chair of the Department of

Anesthesiology), academic affairs (Paul Friedman, M.D., professor of radiology and who had already had the title of associate dean for academic affairs for several years), and scientific affairs (George Palade, M.D.) [David N. Bailey, personal recollections and research].

Having been on the Yale faculty in 1974 when Nobel laureate George Palade, M.D., widely considered to be the "father of modern cell biology" and his wife, Marilyn G. Farquhar, Ph.D., an internationally renowned cell biologist, were recruited from Rockefeller University by Yale dean of medicine Lewis Thomas, Burrow was determined to recruit the couple to UC San Diego School of Medicine in order to improve the basic science stature of the school. In 1990 Palade, age 78, was appointed the first dean for scientific affairs while Farquhar was made the founding head of the Division of Cellular and Molecular Medicine, which would subsequently earn departmental status. As hoped, the recruitment of this dynamic "power couple" was the magnet that subsequently attracted numerous illustrious basic scientists to UC San Diego School of Medicine. On Palade's "watch," many private and public sponsors of biomedical research and training were lured to the school, including the Ludwig Institute for Cancer Research, the Howard Hughes Medical Institute, and the Lucille Markey Foundation. Gerry Burrow considered the recruitment of George Palade and Marilyn Farquhar to be one of the most significant accomplishments of his professional career. As a humorous side-note, because Dean Palade was 78 at the time of his recruitment to UC San Diego, he was ineligible to be appointed a tenured professor since federal law at that time mandated retirement of tenured faculty at age 70. Hence, he was appointed in the "in residence" series to be discussed later [David N. Bailey, personal recollections and research; 23, 24].

Shortly after arrival as dean, Burrow launched national searches for the chairs of the departments of medicine and pathology, resulting in the appointment of both Stephen Wasserman, M.D. as permanent chair of the Department of Medicine and David N. Bailey, M.D. as permanent chair of the Department of Pathology in 1988 [David N. Bailey, personal recollections and research].

The year 1991 saw the creation of the Department of Orthopedics when, as with the Division of Ophthalmology earlier, it was broken out of the Department of Surgery where it had been a division. Wayne Akeson, M.D., head of the division, was appointed the founding chair [David N. Bailey, personal recollections and research].

After serving only four years as vice chancellor and dean, Gerard Burrow heeded the call of his *alma mater*, Yale, to return as its 14th dean of the school of medicine, thereby leaving UC San Diego again without a vice chancellor and dean [David N. Bailey, personal recollections and research , 22].

John F. Alksne (1992 – 1999)

In order to avoid a prolonged period without a vice chancellor and dean during such a critical period of development of the school, Chancellor Atkinson very quickly appointed John Alksne, M.D., founding head of the Division of Neurological Surgery at UC San Diego, to this position. Unlike many of his predecessors Alksne remarkably maintained a clinical practice while serving in this role [David N. Bailey, personal recollections and research]. His numerous chair recruitments were appointments of excellent individuals who were already on the UC San Diego School of Medicine faculty.

One of the first recruitments was the chair of the Department of Pediatrics to replace Michael Kaback, who had resigned to return to the faculty. This was a particularly difficult position to fill since discussions about affiliation of the UC San Diego pediatric service with Children's Hospital of San Diego had been ongoing for many years due to both the seriously declining census of the UC San Diego pediatric inpatient service and the desire of Children's Hospital to become a more academic institution. Despite the synergy that could result from such an affiliation, the prospect of this frightened off some candidates who were perplexed by what the relationship would be between the chair of the Department of Pediatrics at UC San Diego and the Chief of Pediatrics (Physician-in-Chief) at Children's Hospital. (Would they be the same person or two different people?) In 1992, Stanley Mendoza, M.D., professor and head of the Division of Nephrology, was appointed chair of the Department of Pediatrics [David N. Bailey, personal recollections and research; Gabriel Haddad, personal communication, February 15, 2017; John F. Alksne, personal communication, May 24, 2017].

When Robert Katzman stepped down as chair to return to the faculty of the Department of Neurosciences, Dean Alksne appointed Leon Thal, M.D., professor of neurosciences, as chair in 1993. Dr. Thal had come to UC San Diego with Dr. Katzman and was a major figure in the Alzheimer's Disease Research Center [David N. Bailey, personal recollections and research; Doris Trauner, personal communication, February 15, 2017].

When Robert Resnick stepped down as chair to return to the faculty of the Department of Reproductive Medicine and to become School of Medicine Associate Dean for Admissions, Alksne appointed Thomas Moore, M.D., a maternal-fetal medicine specialist and professor of reproductive medicine, as chair in 1995 [David N. Bailey, personal recollections and research; Charles Nager, personal communication, February 15, 2017].

In 1995 Alksne appointed Jerry Schneider, M.D., Professor of Pediatrics, as Dean for Academic Affairs, replacing Paul Friedman, M.D., who returned to the faculty [David N. Bailey, personal recollections and research].

When Wayne Akeson resigned as founding chair of the Department of Orthopedics to return to the faculty Dean Alksne appointed Steven Garfin, internationally renowned spine surgeon and professor of orthopaedic surgery, as chair of the newly renamed Department of Orthopaedic Surgery in 1996 [David N. Bailey, personal recollections and research].

Upon the retirement of Harvey Shapiro as chair of the Department of Anesthesiology Alksne appointed John Drummond, M.D., professor of anesthesiology and chief of the anesthesiology service at the Veterans Affairs San Diego Healthcare System, to be chair in 1997 [David N. Bailey, personal recollections and research; Gerard Manecke, personal communication, February 14, 2017].

In 1997 Elizabeth Barrett-Connor resigned as chair of the Department of Community and Family Medicine to return to the faculty. Robert Kaplan, Ph.D., professor in the department, was appointed interim chair. After two years of service as interim chair, Dr. Kaplan agreed to become permanent chair of the newly renamed Department of Family and Preventive Medicine in 1999 [David N. Bailey, personal recollections and research].

Dean Alksne presided over the formation of the Department of Cellular and Molecular Medicine, previously an autonomous division, in 1999. This was only the second basic-science department in the school. Considerable debate occurred over the naming of the department with Biology maintaining that use of the title "cell biology" would detract from its own program and the Department of Medicine lamenting use of the title "molecular medicine." A compromise was "Cellular and Molecular Medicine," the title subsequently approved by the Academic Senate. Marilyn G. Farquhar, Ph.D., professor and head of the autonomous division, became the founding chair of the department [David N. Bailey, personal recollections and research].

Another notable occurrence on Alksne's "watch" was the opening of the long-awaited campus hospital, the John M. and Sally B. Thornton Hospital and the adjacent Perlman Ambulatory Care Center in 1993. Dean Alksne himself performed the first surgery (a delicate neurosurgery) in the new hospital [25].

A "watershed moment" in Alksne's tenure as dean occurred in 1995-1996 when the UC San Diego Medical Center was projecting more than $25 million of deficit for fiscal year 1996 due to declining hospital census without concomitant reduction in hospital expenses. In response Alksne called in The Hunter Group, a notorious but effective "slash and burn" group who were experts in healthcare system reorganization. The end result was the layoff of several hundred employees and the restructuring of the health system leadership and operational structure. While extraordinarily challenging to do, the health system survived and emerged in much stronger shape as a more efficient ("lean and mean") organization that had embraced discipline and fiscal responsibility [David N. Bailey, personal recollections and research; 26].

David N. Bailey (1999 - 2000)

With little forewarning, in the fall of 1999 John Alksne stepped down as vice chancellor and

dean to return to the faculty and his growing clinical practice. After wide consultation with

faculty, Chancellor Robert Dynes appointed the author, David N. Bailey, M.D., professor and

chair of the Department of Pathology, as the interim vice chancellor and dean. Bailey accepted

with one condition: that he not be a "caretaker" but be allowed to make changes as needed.

The chancellor agreed [David N. Bailey, personal recollections and research].

Bailey began (with chancellorial and UC Office of the President support) by eliminating the

position of healthcare chief executive officer, a construct that had been established by The

Hunter Group almost two years before. This allowed the medical center director once again to

report directly to the vice chancellor and dean without going through an intermediary. Bailey

also decided to push vigorously forward with the long-proposed affiliation agreement with the

Children's Hospital of San Diego (CHSD) and its affiliated medical group, Children's Specialists of

San Diego (CSSD).   Since the CHSD chief executive officer, Blair Sadler, was planning to retire in

one year and since David Bailey assumed that, at best, he would have only one year as interim

vice chancellor and dean, they set a one-year timeline to accomplish this feat. With

determination, the two were able to push the affiliation toward approval of University of

California Regents and the board of trustees of CHSD as well as the board of directors of CSSD.

With the approval of those bodies, inpatient and outpatient pediatric care would be based at

CHSD (later to be known as Rady Children's Hospital of San Diego) except for neonatology

(based at both UC San Diego and CHSD) and ophthalmology. Although smoothing "ruffled

feathers" of some faculty and staff took a few years after the affiliation, the arrangement subsequently would prove to be a "win-win" for both institutions [David N. Bailey, personal recollections and research; 27].

During the year the specialized cancer center designation of the cancer center was threatened due to National Cancer Institute concerns that the faculty were widely dispersed and had no centralized facility. This threat spurred Chancellor Dynes to launch fundraising for what would become the Moores Cancer Center, with its subsequent designation as a comprehensive cancer center. Yet another threat during Bailey's service was the attempt of another prominent southwest cancer institution to lure away the leadership of the Ludwig Institute for Cancer Research (LICR), a UC San Diego affiliated research institute based on the La Jolla campus. By providing LICR with substantially more space, the leadership was retained at UC San Diego [David N. Bailey, personal recollections and research].

While Bailey went to the dean's office in 1999, he appointed Henry C. Powell, M.D., professor and head of the Division of Neuropathology, to serve as the interim chair of the Department of Pathology. Roger Spragg, M.D., professor and vice chair of the Department of Medicine, was appointed interim chair of the Department of Medicine when Steven Wasserman resigned as chair in 2000. Ken Lee Jones, professor of pediatrics and head of the Division of Endocrinology, was appointed interim chair of the Department of Pediatrics when Stanley Mendoza resigned as chair in 2000 [David N. Bailey, personal recollections and research].

At the end of his service as interim vice chancellor and dean, Bailey returned to the chair of the Department of Pathology, looking back upon his year of service by quoting Charles Dickens:

"it was the best of times, it was the worst of times" [David N. Bailey, personal recollections and research; 28].

Edward W. Holmes (2000 – 2006)

After a national search Chancellor Dynes appointed Edward ("Ed") Holmes, M.D. as the vice chancellor for health sciences and dean of the school of medicine in 2000. Holmes was the recently appointed vice chancellor for academic affairs and dean of the school of medicine at Duke University, but these positions did not include oversight of a clinical enterprise, as the position at UC San Diego did. Prior to Duke University Holmes had been senior associate dean for research at Stanford University as well as vice president for translational medicine and clinical research for the Stanford Health System and special counsel to the Stanford president on biomedical research. Earlier he had been chair of the Department of Medicine at the University of Pennsylvania and a Howard Hughes Medical Investigator [29, 30].

One of Holmes's very first actions was to finalize the UC San Diego affiliation agreement with CHSD and CHHC, for which the Regents of the University of California granted formal approval in November 2000 [27]. This set the stage for enhancement of the pediatrics programs at both institutions and became a model for similar affiliations nationwide.

Dean Holmes proved to be a master at chair recruitment. He likened it in some respects to purchase of real estate. First, one had to determine what he/she could afford, then assemble the recruitment package within those resource parameters, and finally present it to finalists for the position. This was in contrast to the customary practice of luring candidates into finalist status and then negotiating back and forth, only to lose the candidate due to inability to provide the package the candidate wanted in the first place. Another unique strategy utilized

by Holmes was the reverse site visit to finalist candidates. He explained that this both flattered

the candidates and gave him an inside look (sometimes quite surprising) at how the candidates

were perceived at their home institutions [David N. Bailey, personal recollections and research].

In 2001 Holmes brought David Bailey, M.D., who had returned to chairing the Department of

Pathology for his 14th year, back into the dean's office in the new position of deputy vice

chancellor for health sciences and dean for faculty and student matters. In these roles Bailey

assisted Holmes in many projects and also provided oversight of academic affairs, faculty

affairs, and medical education. Henry Powell, M.D., Sc.D. was appointed once again as interim

chair of the Department of Pathology in 2001 [David N. Bailey, personal recollections and

research].

The first department chair recruited by Holmes was Kenneth Kaushansky, M.D. as chair of

the Department of Medicine in 2002. Kaushansky had been professor and chief of hematology

at the University of Washington and was well known for his pioneering work on thrombopoietin

[31]. That same year William ("Bill") Bradley, M.D. was appointed chair of the Department of

Radiology in 2002, replacing George Leopold who retired.   Bradley, a renowned expert in

magnetic resonance imaging (MRI) had been director of MRI and radiology research at Long

Beach Memorial Medical Center [32]. Also in 2002 Holmes appointed Joan Heller-Brown, Ph.D.,

professor of pharmacology, to be the interim chair of the Department of Pharmacology, when

Palmer Taylor was appointed dean of the new Skaggs School of Pharmacy and Pharmaceutical

Sciences [David N. Bailey, personal recollections and research]. In 2003 David B. Hoyt, M.D.,

professor of surgery and head of the Division of Trauma, was appointed interim chair of the

Department of Surgery, when "Babs" Moossa returned to the faculty to serve as institutional special liaison for international patients [David N. Bailey, personal recollections and research].

In 2004 and 2005 Dean Holmes appointed a number of new chairs. Steven L. Gonias, M.D., Ph.D. was appointed chair of the Department of Pathology in 2004, replacing Henry C. Powell who collectively had served four years as interim chair of the department. Gonias had been vice chair for research and development in the Department of Pathology at the University of Virginia and associate director for translational research at its cancer center [33]. Also in 2004 Gerard Manecke, M.D., professor of anesthesiology, was appointed interim chair of the Department of Anesthesiology to replace John Drummond, who returned to the faculty [David N. Bailey, personal recollections and research], and in the same year Theodore ("Ted") Ganiats, M.D., professor of family and preventive medicine, was appointed interim chair of the department when Robert Kaplan left to become distinguished professor of health policy and management at UC Los Angeles [David N. Bailey, personal recollections and research].

In 2005, after a national search, Holmes appointed Joan Heller-Brown, interim chair of the Department of Pharmacology, to be its permanent chair. He also appointed Mark Talamini, M.D. as chair of the Department of Surgery. Talamini, professor of surgery at Johns Hopkins, was a pioneer in laparoscopic surgery through natural orifices [David N. Bailey, personal recollections and research]. Also in 2005 Gabriel Haddad, M.D. was appointed chair of the Department of Pediatrics and Physician in Chief of CHHC, replacing Kenneth Lee Jones, who had served in the interim role for an amazing five years. Haddad had been chair of the Department of Pediatrics at Albert Einstein College of Medicine and Pediatrician in Chief at The Children's Hospital at Montefiore Hospital. His research focused on cell and tissue injury in hypoxia [34].

In 2006 Holmes appointed Arno J. ("AJ") Mundt, M.D. as the founding chair of the newly created Department of Radiation Medicine and Applied Sciences. This unit had previously been a hospital department. An internationally recognized radiation oncologist, Dr. Mundt was recruited from the faculty of the University of Chicago [35].

Aside from his expertise in recruiting outstanding department chairs, Holmes recruited other "superstars" to positions in his office. Among these were Thomas McAfee, M.D., recruited in 2002 as the Dean for Clinical Affairs for the UC San Diego Health Sciences and Chief Executive Officer of the UC San Diego Medical Group. McAfee had been associate chief medical officer at UC San Francisco and executive vice president of Brown and Toland Medical Group [36]. Another was the recruitment of Jack Dixon, Ph.D. in 2003 to be the Dean for Scientific Affairs, following George Palade, who had retired in 2001. Dixon had been director of the life sciences institute and chair of the Department of Biological Chemistry at the University of Michigan. From 2001 to 2003 Gordon Gill, M.D., professor of medicine, had served as interim Dean for Scientific Affairs [37]. In 2004 Andrew L. Ries, M.D., professor of medicine, was appointed associate dean (later changed to associate vice chancellor) for academic affairs, and in 2006 Vivian Reznik, M.D., professor of pediatrics, was appointed associate dean (later changed to assistant vice chancellor) for faculty affairs [David N. Bailey, personal recollections and research].

After an immensely successful term as vice chancellor and dean, during which the clinical, educational, and research enterprises flourished, Ed Holmes announced that he would be leaving UC San Diego in the fall of 2006 in order to assume the positions of executive deputy chairman of the Biomedical Research Council of the Agency for Science, Technology and

Research (A-STAR) and executive chairman of the National Medical Research Council of

Singapore [30]. On his watch the institution had matured considerably.

David N. Bailey (2006 – 2007)

In fall 2006 Chancellor Marye Anne Fox appointed David Bailey to serve again as interim vice

chancellor for health sciences and dean of the school of medicine. Because Dean Holmes had

given sufficiently advanced notice of his pending departure, a national search was commenced

before he left. Thus, Bailey's term was less than one year, and, unlike his first term as interim

vice chancellor and dean, he largely served in a "caretaker" role, transitioning out of the interim

role and into his new role as vice chancellor for health affairs and dean of the school of

medicine at UC Irvine one month after the arrival of the next UC San Diego vice chancellor and

dean [David N. Bailey, personal recollections and research].

David A. Brenner (2007 -)

Having gone through seven permanent vice chancellor/deans and five interim ones (one of

whom served twice) in 43 years, the school had garnered enough stature and resources for the

right leader to "ride the wave" and to take the school into its prime. After a national search,

Chancellor Fox appointed David Brenner, M.D., the Samuel Bard Professor and Chair of the

Department of Medicine at Columbia University, Physician-in-chief of New York Presbyterian

Hospital/Columbia and a renowned research gastroenterologist, as the next vice chancellor and

dean and, as of this time, the longest serving individual in that position. Brenner was well

acquainted with UC San Diego because in 1985 he had completed a gastroenterology fellowship

at UC San Diego and had joined the faculty as a PEW Scholar and clinical investigator, leaving in

1992 to become professor and chief of the Division of Digestive Disease and Nutrition at the University of North Carolina [David N. Bailey, personal recollections and research; 14].

From almost the moment that he took office (February 1, 2007), Brenner set upon a vigorous agenda of recruiting and building, often pushing the envelope to its very limits [David N. Bailey, personal recollections and research]. As he described himself: "…I am aggressive programmatically and have leveraged us a lot. I know where I want to go….I came back here to do something amazing, and I don't think long term we would be a great institution if we didn't keep pushing and doing new things" [39].

A few months after he arrived, Leon Thal, the chair of the Department of Neurosciences, was killed in a plane accident. Brenner called Doris Trauner, M.D., professor and head of the Division of Pediatric Neurology, into service as interim chair for a second time (2007 – 2009). In 2008 he made Gerard Manecke, M.D., interim chair of the Department of Anesthesiology, its permanent chair. That same year saw two founding department chairs step down to return to the faculty: Stuart Brown, M.D., chair of Ophthalmology and Marilyn Farquhar, Ph.D., chair of Cellular and Molecular Medicine. Brenner appointed Robert Weinreb, M.D., professor of ophthalmology, as it chair and Donald Cleveland, Ph.D., professor of cellular and molecular medicine, as its chair [David N. Bailey, personal recollections and research].

After a lengthy national search William Mobley, M.D., Ph.D., the John E. Cahill Family Professor in the Department of Neurology and Neurological Sciences and founding Director of the Neuroscience Institute at Stanford University, was appointed chair of the Department of Neurosciences in 2009 [40]. In 2010 Kenneth Kaushansky, M.D. left as chair of the Department of Medicine to become dean at Stony Brook University School of Medicine, and Wolfgang Dillmann, M.D., professor of medicine/endocrinology and metabolism, was appointed interim chair of the department, subsequently being made permanent chair in 2012 [David N. Bailey, personal recollections and research].

In 2011 Bess Marcus, Ph.D., professor of psychiatry and human behavior and community health at Brown University, was appointed chair of the once again renamed Department of Family Medicine and Public Health, replacing Theodore Ganiats, M.D. who had earned the dubious distinction of being the longest serving interim chair (seven years) [David N. Bailey, personal recollections and research]!

In 2013 Emergency Medicine, a hospital department for many years, was granted status as an academic department of the school of medicine. Theodore ("Ted") Chan, M.D., professor of medicine/emergency medicine, was appointed as its founding chair [David N. Bailey, personal recollections and research]. In the same year Mark Talamini, M.D. left UC San Diego to become chair of the Department of Surgery at Stony Brook, having been recruited away by its new dean and his former chair colleague, Kenneth Kaushansky. Brenner then appointed Christopher Kane, M.D., professor of surgery and head of the Division of Urology, as interim chair of the Department of Surgery [David N. Bailey, personal recollections and research].

After an amazing run of 36 years as chair of the Department of Psychiatry, Lewis Judd, M.D. retired in 2014, and Igor Grant, M.D., professor and executive vice chair of the department, was appointed permanent chair [David N. Bailey, personal recollections and research; 41]. That same year Charles Nager, M.D., professor of reproductive medicine, was appointed chair when incumbent Thomas Moore, M.D. was appointed Dean for Clinical Affairs and Chief Executive Officer of the Medical Group, to succeed Thomas McAfee, M.D., who had announced his departure to become Chief Executive Officer of the Keck Medicine of USC Foundation, a position which unfortunately he did not assume due to being killed by elephants while on a safari trip in Africa [David N. Bailey, personal recollections and research; 42]!

In 2015 the Division of Dermatology in the Department of Medicine was granted academic department status with Richard Gallo, M.D., head of the division, being appointed its founding chair [David N. Bailey, personal recollections and research].   In the same year Bryan Clary, M.D., professor and chief of hepatobiliary surgery at Duke University, was appointed chair of the Department of Surgery and Surgeon-in-Chief for the UC San Diego Health System [David N. Bailey, personal recollections and research; 43]. Finally, in 2015, Alexander Norbash, M.D., professor and chair of the Department of Radiology at Boston University and an esteemed interventional neuroradiologist, was appointed chair of the Department of Radiology when William Bradley, M.D. retired [David N. Bailey, personal recollections and research; 44].

In 2016 William Mobley, M.D. stepped down as chair of the Department of Neurosciences, becoming associate dean for neurosciences initiatives, and James Brewer, M.D., Professor of Neurosciences, was appointed interim chair [David N. Bailey, personal recollections and research].

In 2017 the Division of Urology in the Department of Surgery was granted academic department status with Christopher Kane, M.D., professor and head of the division, being appointed its founding chair. That action made 17 academic departments overall in the school of medicine, almost double the nine departments when the school was founded (medicine, neurosciences, obstetrics & gynecology, pathology, pediatrics, preventive medicine, psychiatry, radiology, and surgery) [David N. Bailey, personal recollections and research].

Although from the above it might seem that David Brenner spent most of his time creating new departments and recruiting chairs, he recruited a number of other significant positions. In 2010 he appointed Maria Savoia, M.D., a nationally renowned educator, as dean for medical education. Savoia, professor of medicine and an infectious diseases specialist, had previously been associate dean for curriculum and student affairs (1990 – 2003) and then, under vice chancellor and dean Holmes, had become vice-dean for medical education [David N. Bailey, personal recollections and research]. In the same year (2010) Brenner appointed Gary Firestein, M.D., professor and head of the Division of Rheumatology, Allergy, and Immunology, as dean for translational medicine and director of the Clinical and Translational Research Institute. As previously noted, in 2014 Brenner appointed Thomas Moore, M.D. to be dean for clinical affairs and chief executive officer of the Medical Group [David N. Bailey, personal recollections and research]. In 2017, Brenner created a new position, Associate Vice Chancellor whose role included service as the Health Sciences Chief Academic Officer, and, after a national search, he appointed to this post Douglas Ziedonis, M.D., M.P.H., professor and chair of the University of Massachusetts Department of Psychiatry, President of the University of Massachusetts Behavioral Health Services, and an internationally renowned expert in co-occurring mental illness and addiction [David N. Bailey, personal recollections and research; 45]. Also in 2017, Bess Marcus, Chair of the Department of Family Medicine and Public Health was recruited to be Dean of the School of Public Health at Brown University, and Cheryl Anderson, Ph.D., associate professor of Family Medicine and Public Health, was appointed interim chair [David N. Bailey, personal recollections and research].

In 2018 the Department of Reproductive Medicine was renamed the Department of Obstetrics, Gynecology, and Reproductive Sciences. In the same year interim chair James Brewer was named permanent chair of the Department of Neurosciences, and Ruth Waterman, Associate Professor of Anesthesiology, was named interim chair of the Department of Anesthesiology when Gerard Manecke returned to the faculty [David N. Bailey, personal recollections and research].

In addition to his recruitment of people who held major administrative posts, Brenner recruited several dozen other prominent well-known individuals who are internationally renowned in their fields of research. Such recruitments were undoubtedly aided by the fact that Brenner himself has maintained an active extramurally funded research program. In fact, Brenner stated that "I had cachet with the scientists because I am a funded investigator" [39].

Although the affiliation agreement between UC San Diego, Rady Children's Hospital of San Diego (RCHSD), and the Children's Specialists of San Diego (CSSD) had been approved by the UC Regents in November 2000, the CSSD physicians continued to be only voluntary faculty at UC San Diego. Unfortunately this created the perception of "classes" of faculty between the two institutions. On Brenner's watch in 2009, with the generous financial support of RCHSD and the concurrence of UC San Diego faculty, CSSD faculty were allowed to decide whether or not to accept salaried faculty appointments at UC San Diego or to remain CSSD employees. In the end, about 120 CSSD faculty in multiple specialties moved to salaried UC San Diego faculty status. Accordingly, the affiliation was now "complete" in the strictest sense of the word (46).

Aside from his recruitment talents, Brenner has been a fundraiser *extraordinaire*! Among his numerous accomplishments have been securing many multi-million dollar donations from Joan and Irwin Jacobs, T. Denny Sanford, Donald and Darlene Shiley, Lisa and Steve Altman, and Richard and Maria Sulpizio, among others, whose collective generosity made possible a vast number of clinical and research facilities and programs to be described later. This also gave Brenner the distinction of being a "master builder," in both the literal and the figurative sense [David N. Bailey, personal recollections and research]. On his watch, employment on the La Jolla campus of the health sciences grew from 1,500 to more than 8,000 [39].

A Change in the Model

Given the increased responsibilities and complexities of the vice chancellorship, the position of vice chancellorship for health sciences and dean of the school of medicine was split in 2018 (47). In fact, UC Irvine and UC Davis had already done this. The need for such split was accentuated by the development of additional health sciences professional schools at these campuses, which logically wanted to report to the vice chancellor instead of the dean of the school of medicine. Indeed, by 2018, a proposal for a school of public health in UC San Diego health sciences was on the drawing board. In 2018, Chancellor Khosla appointed Steven Garfin, M.D., Chair of the Department of Orthopaedic Surgery, as the interim dean, and Reid Abrams, M.D. was appointed interim chair of the Department of Orthopaedic Surgery.

In a little more than fifty years the UC San Diego School of Medicine had not only caught the wave but was riding it for all it was worth!

References

1. In Memoriam: John S. O'Brien: 1934-2001, UC San Diego Health Sciences Press Release, http://ucsdnews.ucsd.edu/archive/newsrel/health/obrien.htm

2. UC San Diego Department of Medicine website, http://med.ucsd.edu.

3. Oral History of Robert Hamburger, April 20, 2000, UCSD Oral Histories. Special Collection & Archives, U John Moxley Resigned as Vice Chancellor for Health Sciences and Dean of School of Medicine, September 22, 1980, University Communications & Public Relations Materials: News Releases. Special Collections & Archives, UC San Diego Library.

4. Physicians for Reproductive Health: Kenneth J. Ryan, M.D., https://prh.org/provider-voices/kenneth-j-ryan-md-memorial-program/programs-kenneth-j-ryan-md/

5. Obituary: Samuel S.C. Yen, 1927 – 2006, International Figure in Reproductive Medicine. UC San Diego News Release, January 3, 2007, http://ucsdnews.ucsd.edu/archive/newsrel/health/yen07.asp

6. John Moxley Resigned as Vice Chancellor for Health Sciences and Dean of School of Medicine, September 22, 1980, University Communications & Public Relations Materials: News Releases. Special Collections & Archives, UC San Diego Library.

7. Two Receptions Will Be Given in Honor of Dr. John H. Moxley III and Mrs. Moxley, September 6, 1973, University Communications & Public Relations Materials: News Releases. Special Collections & Archives, UC San Diego Library.

8. In Memoriam: Helen M. Ranney, M.D., UC San Diego Health News Release, April 8, 2010, https://health.ucsd.edu/news/2010/Pages/4-8-obit-ranney.aspx

9. Doris A. Howell, M.D., Hospice and Pediatric Oncology Expert, Women's Health Advocate, Women's International Center Biographies, http://www.wic.org/bio/dhowell.htm

10. In Memoriam: Colin M. Bloor, Council of University of California Emeriti Associations, September 2010, http://cucea.ucsd.edu/reports/InMemorianColinBloor.htm

11. Lewis Judd to Step Down After 36 Years as Chair of Department of Psychiatry, June 13, 2013, University Communications & Public Relations Materials: News Releases. Special Collections & Archives, UC San Diego Library.

12. Society of Abdominal Radiology Past Presidents: Robert N. Berk, MD, http://www.abdominalradiology.org/general/custom.asp?page=SGRPastPresidents

13. NA Anderson: Improbable Venture: A History of the University of California, San Diego. The UCSD Press, La Jolla, California, 1993, pp 153-180.

14. Dr. Marvin R. Dunn, 71, Respected Advocate for New Doctors, Chicago Tribune, August 3, 2003.

15. Hollingsworth is New Med Dean. The Daily Guardian, University of California, San Diego, October 17, 1980.

16. RG Petersdorf and PB Beeson: Fever of unexplained origin: report on 100 cases. Medicine 40: 1 – 30 (1961.

17. LK Altman: Robert Petersdorf, 80, Major Force in U.S. Medicine Dies, *New York Times*, October 6, 2006.

18. D. Kain: Dr. Robert Katzman, Pioneering Alzheimer's Disease Expert, Dies, September 18, 2008, http://ucsdnews.ucsd.edu/archive/newsrel/health/09-08Katzman.asp

19. MM Kaback: Michael Kaback: people and places. *Genetics in Medicine* 16: 981 (2014).

20. I Oransky: Robert Petersdorf – Obituary. *The Lancet* 368: 1764 (2006).

21. In Memoriam – Wayne Akeson, M.D., Office of the Vice Chancellor for Health Sciences Communication, November 8, 2016.

22. L Landsberg: Gerard N. Burrow, M.D., 1933 – 2013, *Transactions of the American Clinical and Climatological Association* 126: LXXXII – LXXXIV

23. George Palade, UC San Diego Department of Cellular and Molecular Medicine Website, https://healthsciences.ucsd.edu/som/cmm/about/george-palade/Pages/default.aspx

24. L Franz: Nobel Laureate, "Father of Modern Cell Biology," Dies at Age 95, UC San Diego News Center, October 10, 2008.

25. UC San Diego Health: About Us – Our History, https://health.ucsd.edu/about/pages/history.aspx

26. UC San Diego Annual Financial Report 1996: The Mission Made Possible, http://annualreport.ucsd.edu/1996/hlthsci.html

27. Regents Approve Efforts to Unite UCSD Pediatrics and Children's Hospital, November 16, 2000, http://ucsdnews.ucsd.edu/archive/newsrel/health/ucsdchildrens.htm

28. C. Dickens: A Tale of Two Cities, 1859.

29. Edward Holmes, M.D. Selected as New Vice Chancellor for Health Sciences, July 20, 2000. University Communications & Public Relations Materials: News Releases. Special Collections & Archives, UC San Diego Library.

30. Edward W. Holmes, M.D., The Lowy Medical Research Institute, http://www.lmri.net/edward-w-holmes-m-d/

31. UCSD Announces New Chair of Medicine, January 10, 2002, University Communications & Public Relations Materials: News Releases. Special Collections & Archives, UC San Diego Library.

32. National MRI Expert Named New Chair of UCSD Department of Radiology, May 14, 2002. University Communications & Public Relations Materials: News Releases. Special Collections & Archives, UC San Diego Library.

33. UCSD Names Steven L. Gonias New Chair of Pathology, April 16, 2004. University Communications & Public Relations Materials: News Releases. Special Collections & Archives, UC San Diego Library.

34. Rady Children's Hospital of San Diego Website, Gabriel Haddad, M.D. http://www.rchsd.org/doctors/gabriel-haddad-md/

35. UC San Diego Health Sciences Department of Radiation Medicine and Applied Sciences Website, Arno J. Mundt, M.D., http://healthsciences.ucsd.edu/som/radiation-medicine/people/faculty/pages/arno-mundt.aspx

36. L Ridgeway: McAfee Named CEO of New Keck Medicine of USC Foundation, USC News, August 7, 2013, https://news.usc.edu/53868/mcafee-named-ceo-of-new-keck-medicine-of-usc-medical-foundation/

37. Office of the Vice Chancellor – Health Sciences: Dean for Scientific Affairs, December 17, 2001, http://adminrecords.ucsd.edu/notices/2002/2002-12-17-1.html

38. Distinguished Gastroenterologist Named UC San Diego Vice Chancellor for Health Sciences, Dean of Medical School, January 18, 2007, University Communications & Public Relations Materials: News Releases. Special Collections & Archives, UC San Diego Library.

39. G Robbins: "Empire Builder" Has UCSD Health on the Rise, *San Diego Union-Tribune*, August 21, 2015.

40. UC San Diego Department of Neurosciences Website, William Mobley, M.D., Ph.D., https://neurosciences.ucsd.edu/faculty/pages/william-mobley.aspx

41. Lewis Judd to Step Down After 36 Years as chair of Department of Psychiatry, June 13, 2013, University Communications & Public Relations Materials: News Releases. Special Collections & Archives, UC San Diego Library.

42. L Ridgeway: McAfee Named CEO of New Keck Medicine of USC Foundation, USC News, August 7, 2013, https://news.usc.edu/53868/mcafee-named-ceo-of-new-keck-medicine-of-usc-medical-foundation

43. Institute of Engineering in Medicine: Bryan M. Clary, https://iem.ucsd.edu/people/profiles/bryan_clary.html

44. Institute of Engineering in Medicine, Alexander Norbash, https://iem.ucsd.edu/people/profiles/alexander_norbash.html

45. Douglas M. Ziedonis, http://neurosciencecme.com/cmea_popup_faculty.asp?ID=307

46. UCSD/RCHSD Affiliation Agreements Review. Audit Project 2011-25.

47. Appointment for Vice Chancellor – Health Sciences David A. Brenner, M.D. and Interim Dean – School of Medicine Steven Garfin, M.D. http://adminrecords.ucsd.edu/notices/2018/2018-4-2-5.html

Chapter 6

The Medical Center and Its Evolution

You may wonder why the history of a school of medicine would contain a chapter on the medical center. Aside from the need for a faculty practice and clinical teaching site, in modern-day academic medicine, the medical center (aka "health system") is the financial "engine" of the school of medicine, providing funding both "above the line" (i.e., directly to faculty for services rendered) and "below the line" (i.e., transfers to the school), depending upon the configuration of the academic enterprise. This chapter will track the history of the UC San Diego Medical Center.

The Early Days: Operating a County-Owned Facility (1966 – 1981)

In 1963 the 600-bed county hospital was completed in the Hillcrest section of San Diego at a cost of $11.5 million for both building and equipment. Currently still in use, this facility was a "rebuild" adjacent to the site of the first official three-story "county hospital" constructed in 1903-04 for $60,000 [1, 2]. Three years later (1966) UC San Diego assumed the operation of the new facility as its primary clinical teaching site (University Hospital of San Diego County) for the planned new medical school with private patients being allowed to use the facility for the first time. Under the arrangement with the County of San Diego, UC San Diego would be ceded parcels of land on which teaching and research functions would be developed with about 31 acres available immediately and an additional 12.5 acres (including space at Vauclain Point) being transferred if needed in the future. It was proposed that changes in the hospital would be "evolutionary rather than revolutionary." UC San Diego would be responsible for all activities except for determination of patient eligibility, processing of accounts receivable, community mental health activities, laundry, power plant, and maintenance department. Staff in those areas would continue to be county employees. Others who had attained permanent civil service status would be given the opportunity of transferring to UC San Diego or remaining with the county. Temporary, provisional, interim, and unclassified employees would be transferred to UC San Diego. Those who elected to remain with the county would be transferred to UC San Diego when promoted or advanced. Medical policies for the hospital would be under the direction of then medical school dean Joseph Stokes while business operations would be overseen by the UC San Diego Vice Chancellor for Business and Finance, Robert Biron. The hospital administrator would continue to be A.F. Crumley, M.D. [1, 3, 4].

In that same year (1966) Richard A. Lockwood, M.D. was appointed director of the hospital and clinics, reporting directly to the UC San Diego Chancellor Galbraith. Lockwood had been recruited in 1965 as an assistant to Dean Stokes for hospitals and institutions. He had been assistant clinical professor of surgery at UC Los Angeles and then a consultant to the University of Hawaii, helping in the planning of its two-year biomedical program [5].

In 1972 Chancellor William McElroy hired Sheldon King as the director of the hospital. King had been an assistant professor at Albert Einstein College of Medicine [David N. Bailey, personal recollections and research; 6]. Under Director King several major construction projects occurred. In 1973 the new emergency services department and the first and only regional burn center opened, followed by a federally sponsored General Clinical Research Center in 1974 [1]. In 1976 the regional trauma center opened, and groundbreaking for the outpatient center in Hillcrest occurred. In 1978 the UC San Diego Theodore Gildred Cancer

Center was founded and was designated as a specialized cancer by the National Cancer Institute [7]. John Mendelsohn, M.D., associate professor of medicine, was appointed the first director [8]. The center was named for a developer who had died of cancer in 1967 [9]. In the same year the clinical teaching facility (a misnomer since it contained research laboratories and offices for faculty based at the medical center) was completed [Gary Matthews, personal communication, March 17, 2017].

In 1981 groundbreaking for the Theodore Gildred Cancer Center building and a medical library occurred. The total project cost was $6 million, of which $3.1 million was acquired from the National Institutes of Health, $959,000 from the State of California for the library, and the rest from philanthropy, with the lead gift being from the Gildred Foundation of San Diego. The facility was a four-story building with 34,000 asf and an adjacent two-story medical library [1, 8, 10].

University-Owned But Still Hillcrest-Based (1981 – 1991)

Having operated the county medical center for 15 years, in 1981 the University of California purchased both the hospital and the adjacent county mental health facility for $17 million with annual county support of $2.3 million [David N. Bailey, personal recollections and research; 1]. In that same year director Sheldon King left to become president of the Stanford University Medical Center. Deputy director Vincent Wayne was appointed acting director [11].

In 1982 Robert Erra, senior vice president of Scripps Clinic and Research Foundation, was appointed director by Vice Chancellor and Dean Robert Petersdorf. At that time the hospital director started reporting to the vice chancellor/dean for clinical activities and to the chancellor via the vice chancellor/dean for financial and management matters. This was an important change allowing the school of medicine to have authority over the medical center. Previous directors had reported exclusively to the chancellor [David N. Bailey, personal recollections and research]. Erra was known to be a financial "guru," who was reputed to have negotiated among the first million-dollar contracts for baseball players (a paltry sum by today's standards) [David N. Bailey, personal recollections and research; 11]. Although successful as the director, Erra was lured into the private sector after little more than a year on the job. Petersdorf then appointed Michael Stringer, associate director, to be the interim director, and in 1984 Petersdorf appointed Stringer as the permanent director [David N. Bailey, personal recollections and research; 6].

From the founding of the school of medicine a campus hospital had been envisioned, but financial and political considerations kept that from moving forward until 1988, when, with the vigorous support of Chancellor Richard C. Atkinson and under the guidance of Vice Chancellor and Dean Gerard Burrow, the UC Regents by a narrow vote approved the construction of an east-campus "satellite medical facility," so-called in order to emphasize to the community that this entity was to be merely a "supplement" to the medical center in Hillcrest and not a threat to other hospitals nearby. (The inclusion of an emergency department in the structure strongly suggested that this was just the beginning of the evolution of a major medical center on the university's east campus). As Chancellor Atkinson told the Regents: "UCSD could not be a great university without a great medical school, and we could not have a great medical school without a campus hospital. If the Regents do not vote to approve the project, I will resign as chancellor" [12]. At that meeting Burrow explained that 120 licensed beds (108 general medical-surgical beds and 12 critical care beds) would be transferred from the Hillcrest facility, and the two structures would be operated under a common license and management. An ambulatory care center would be built adjacent to the new hospital. Services would be rationalized between the two campuses with trauma, burn, transplantation, and the neonatology intensive care unit to remain at Hillcrest. The total number of licensed beds would decrease to 327 due to building improvements (e.g., conversion of some multi-bed units in Hillcrest to single-bed units). Burrow also emphasized that, while university hospitals on average had 1,500 asf per bed, UC San Diego had only 778! Even community hospitals had more (1,000 asf per bed). As he put it, "the proposed campus hospital is absolutely vital to the academic future of the medical school, providing basic researchers opportunities to work closely with clinicians." The estimated cost was $74.1 million, with a $5 million naming gift from John M and Sally B Thornton and the rest funded largely through debt-service and additional fundraising. The concept was that the new medical center would draw a better patient sponsorship mix, which would help to support the Hillcrest facility [David N. Bailey, personal recollections and research; 13 – 15].

The East Campus Emerges (1991 – 2004)

Three years later (1991), while Gerard Burrow was still vice chancellor and dean, groundbreaking for the Thornton Hospital and the adjoining Edith and William M Perlman Ambulatory Care Center occurred. The latter cost $8 million with a naming gift coming from the Perlman family [1]. In the same year the main building of the Shiley Eye Institute was opened, named in recognition of the $1 million leadership gift from Donald and Darlene Shiley. Additional support was provided by the National Eye Institute and the Conrad Hilton

Foundation, each of which contributed $500,000. The facility contained 34,144 asf for patient care, research, classrooms, conference rooms, and offices [16]. While most construction activity at this time was focused on development of the east campus, the Hillcrest campus received attention when a new bed tower was "topped off" in 1991 [1].

Finally, in 1993, the long-awaited opening of the Thornton Hospital occurred with the first surgery being performed by the new vice chancellor and dean John Alksne, a neurosurgeon [1] and the first patient being none other than Chancellor Atkinson himself [12]! Despite the appeal of having a full-fledged university medical center in La Jolla, the first several years saw a meager average daily inpatient census (20 – 30 patients only). Rival hospitals, that felt threatened by the Thornton Hospital (particularly since it had an emergency department), gloated over the poor census. Fortunately, after a few more years, the census began to rise dramatically [David N. Bailey, personal recollections and research].

In 1994 the Bannister Family House was opened on the Hillcrest campus. This facility, made possible by the Ralph Bannister family, provided housing for families of patients who were receiving long-term care and wanted to stay near their family member [7]. In 1995 the Anne and Abraham Ratner Eye Center was opened on the east campus adjacent to the Shiley Eye Center thanks to the generosity of the Ratner family [7].

Despite considerable progress in the medical center, calamity struck. As previously noted, in 1995 - 1996, the medical center found itself projecting an operating deficit of $25 million (a large number now but even more disturbing at that time). With support from the chancellor, the vice chancellor/dean John Alksne called in The Hunter Group, an effective "slash and burn" group known for its tough approach to turning financial operations around. Over the next tension-filled two years, the medical center laid off numerous employees, departments trimmed their budgets, and the medical center restructured its operations. During this period (1997) director Michael Stringer resigned, and vice chancellor and dean Alksne appointed Sumiyo ("Sumi") Kastelic, who had been chief operating officer of the medical center since 1990, as director [17]. A chief financial officer, David Sakai, was recruited to oversee the financial operations of the health system, and a chief executive officer for the health system, Kent Sherwood, was recruited from Sutter Healthcare to oversee the medical center and medical group [David N. Bailey, personal recollections and research]. Subsequently in 1999, as previously related in chapter 5, interim vice chancellor and dean David Bailey eliminated the latter position, thus allowing the medical center director, the faculty medical group, and the chief financial officer, to report directly to the vice chancellor and dean [David N. Bailey, personal recollections and research].

In 2001, shortly after arrival of vice chancellor and dean Edward ("Ed") Holmes, the UC San Diego Cancer Center received its long-awaited National Cancer Institute (NCI) designation as a comprehensive cancer center. As noted in chapter 5, the cancer center had been threatened with loss of NCI designation during a 1999-2000 site visit due to lack of space for centralizing research and patient care. However, this was warded off by zealous lobbying on the part of Chancellor Dynes and Vice Chancellor Holmes and by a vigorous fundraising effort to build a new center that would house clinical care and research. By 2000 – 2001, $47 million in private support had been raised with a goal of $75 million for construction and $25 million to support clinical care initiatives in the facility. A naming gift of $20 million was provided by John and

Rebecca Moores with a lead gift of $15 million from Jerome and Miriam Katzin. The building, to be located on the east campus, would contain 270,000 asf of research space, outpatient services, and community education and outreach [David N. Bailey, personal recollections and research; 18, 19].

When director Sumi Kastelic retired in 2002, Holmes recruited Richard Liekweg to be the new medical center chief executive officer. Liekweg had been the chief executive officer of the Durham Regional Hospital, a part of the Duke University Health System [20].

Transformational Changes on the East Campus: "Riding the Wave" (2004 – 2017)

The year 2004 saw the start of additional major expansion of the east campus medical center. In that year both the Joan and Irwin Jacobs Retina Center and the Hamilton Glaucoma Center were opened as a part of the Shiley Eye Center [7]. Also in that year the University of California Regents approved the construction of the long-awaited cardiovascular center, which would include expansion of the adjoining Thornton Hospital [21].

After eight years of planning and more than two years of construction, the Rebecca and John Moores Cancer Center opened in 2005 [22]. Because of the magnitude of construction (both clinical buildings and research buildings, to be described in another chapter) that occurred under Ed Holmes, he was dubbed the "multi-crane dean," seemingly always having one project in planning and one under construction throughout his administration (2000 – 2006) [David N. Bailey, personal recollections and research].

That said, the tenure of Vice Chancellor and Dean Brenner heralded a magnitude of construction that was unparalleled in the history of the school [David N. Bailey, personal recollections and research]. In 2007, shortly after Brenner's arrival, groundbreaking for the Sulpizio Family Cardiovascular Center occurred. The center, named for Richard and Maria ("Gaby") Sulpizio who had contributed $10 million, would be a four-story building that would unify ambulatory, clinical, and inpatient heart and stroke care in one location. A total of $30 million (including the Sulpizio gift) had been raised. As previously noted, it would also add space to the adjoining Thornton Hospital, including its emergency department [23].

The most ambitious project in the history of UC San Diego Health was launched that same year (2007) when the University of California Regents approved planning for the addition of 125 - 150 new beds as an extension of the Thornton Hospital on the east campus [24].

In both 2008 and 2010 Donald and Darlene Shiley again provided gifts to add additional wings to the main building of the Shiley Eye Center [7]. In 2009 the Radiation Oncology PET/CT Center was opened near the Moores Cancer Center [Arno J. Mundt, personal communication, July 4, 2017]. In 2010 Brenner appointed Thomas ("Tom") Jackiewicz to be the chief executive officer of the medical center when Richard Liekweg left to become chief executive officer of Washington University's Barnes Hospital. Jackiewicz had served as Ed Holmes's chief of staff when he was chair of the Department of Medicine at University of Pennsylvania and had been recruited to UC San Diego by Holmes in 2001 as his chief of staff, later becoming associate vice chancellor and chief financial officer [David N. Bailey, personal recollections and research; 25].

In 2010 UC San Diego received its clinical and translational science award of $37.2 million from the National Institutes of Health National Center for Advancing Translational Science. In that same year the University of California Regents approved the budget and financing for the

$269 million externally financed Clinical and Translational Research Institute building to be constructed on the east campus, and Gary Firestein, M.D. became director of the institute [26, 27].

Advancing the evolution of the east campus, in 2010, Joan and Irwin Jacobs pledged $75 million (the largest gift in the history of the UC San Diego Health Sciences) to build the Jacobs Medical Center on the east campus, thereby expanding the vision of the 2007 UC Regents approval of additional beds. The Jacobs Medical Center would include a ten-story 490,000 asf facility of 245 patient beds with three new hospitals: cancer hospital, hospital for women and infants, and hospital for advanced surgery [28].

The year 2011 saw the opening of several new buildings on the health sciences east campus. The Center for Advanced Laboratory Medicine (CALM), a 90,000 asf facility housing state-of-the-art clinical laboratories, was opened in leased space on Campus Point Drive. This center, the vision of Department of Pathology Chair, Steven Gonias, M.D., Ph.D., would serve as a modern diagnostic reference laboratory for UC San Diego [David N. Bailey, personal recollections and research; 1, 7]. The East Campus Office Building, a facility providing offices for faculty and staff working on the east campus, and the Sulpizio Cardiovascular Center, San Diego's first dedicated cardiovascular center, were both opened in 2011 [1]. The $227 million cardiovascular center was funded with $129.9 million in external financing, $38 million in gifts, $21.7 million in hospital reserves, and $37.7 million from capitalized leases [29]. Also, in 2011, Steve and Lisa Altman provided a $10 million naming gift for the Clinical and Translational Research Institute [30].

In 2012 Tom Jackiewicz left UC San Diego to become senior vice president and chief executive officer for the University of Southern California Health System. David Brenner appointed Paul Viviano as chief executive officer for the UC San Diego Health System. Viviano had been chairman of the board and the chief executive officer of Alliance Healthcare and, before that, he had been president and chief executive officer for University of Southern California University Hospital and the Norris Cancer Hospital [31].

Viviano's arrival was marked with several landmark events: the groundbreaking for the Jacobs Medical Center [1] in 2012 and a $100 million pledge from T. Denny Sanford for a stem cell center in 2013 [1]. In 2015, in recognition of the many contributions of the Shileys to the eye center, which had several named components, it was renamed the Donald P. and Darlene V. Shiley Eye Institute [32].

Despite the excitement of UC San Diego Health System expansion, Viviano decided to leave the institution in 2015 to become director of the Children's Hospital of Los Angeles, and David Brenner appointed Patty Maysent, chief strategy officer and chief of staff for UC San Diego Health System, as the interim chief executive officer [33]. In the same year UC San Diego School of Medicine received its renewal of the clinical and translational science award for $52 million (a $15 million increase from the 2010 award) [34].

In 2016 Brenner appointed Patty Maysent the permanent chief executive officer for UC San Diego Health. Maysent, a former Olympic-trained swimmer, hit the ground running. In that year both the Altman Clinical and Translational Research Institute and the long-awaited, transformational Jacobs Medical Center opened [1]. Joan and Irwin Jacobs contributed an additional $25 million to provide a total gift of $100 million with the end result being a nearly $1 billion facility of 509,500 asf with four pavilions: the Thornton Pavilion (original Thornton Hospital), the Rady Pavilion for Women and Infants (so named for a gift from the Ernest Rady family), the Pauline and Stanley Foster Pavilion for Cancer Care (named for a gift from the Foster family), and the A. Vassiliadis Family Pavilion for Advanced Surgery (named for a gift from the Vasiliades family). The majority of rooms featured floor to ceiling windows with panoramic views and i-pad controlled environments with Apple television for entertainment. The i-pads also permitted patients to obtain up-to-date information on their healthcare results and providers. A neonatal intensive care unit, birth center, and labor and delivery unit were also part of the new facility as well as the first intraoperative computerized tomography (CT) and magnetic resonance imaging (MRI) units in San Diego [David N. Bailey, personal recollections and research; 35].

In 2016, in order to accommodate the increased volume of outpatient surgery, construction of the UC San Diego Outpatient Pavilion on the east campus was started. This $140 million, 140,000 gsf facility consolidated outpatient surgical services and integrated them with diagnostics and physical therapy on the east campus neighborhood (ambulatory surgery, outpatient imaging, physical therapy, disease-specific clinics focusing on pain, urology, musculoskeletal care, breast care, and infusion). Opened in March 2018, the facility was named the Koman Family Outpatient Pavilion in honor of Bill and Amy Koman and family in recognition of their generosity and dedication to advancing healthcare in San Diego [36]. Finally, planning for a Center for Novel Therapeutics was launched in 2017. This 110,000 gsf three-story facility would have both wet and dry laboratories, research support space, bioengineering core facilities, human subject assessment space, a lecture hall, and offices and would be in close proximity to the Moores Cancer Center. It would facilitate transition of therapies into the clinical arena [37].

Although the UC San Diego Health System had dramatically increased its clinical space under Brenner, its expansion of clinics into the community was also nothing short of spectacular! A list of clinics and practice sites is contained in the Appendix to this book. In addition, UC San Diego Health expanded its reach by creating clinics in a new model under the purview of the Clinical Practice Organization with physicians and staff being employed directly by this entity. These clinics (currently under development) are not listed in the Appendix [David N. Bailey, personal recollections and research].

In the clinical arena UC School of Medicine was indeed riding the wave!

References

1. UC San Diego Health: About Us – Our History, https://health.ucsd.edu/about/pages/history.aspx
2. M. Kelley: First Annual Report of the San Diego County Hospital and Poor Farm to the Board of Supervisors, for the Year Ending June 30, 1889. *Journal of San Diego History* 48 (4), Fall 2002.
3. County Hospital Transferred to UCSD School of Medicine, March 17, 1965, University Communications & Public Relations Materials: News Releases. Special Collections & Archives, UC San Diego Library.
4. Final Transfer of County Hospital, June 30, 1966, University Communications & Public Relations Materials: News Releases. Special Collections & Archives, UC San Diego Library.
5. Livingston & Lockwood Join School of Medicine Staff, June 24, 1965, University Communications & Public Relations Materials: News Releases. Special Collections &De Archives, UC San Diego Library.
6. N.A. Anderson. An Improbable Venture: A History of the University of California, San Diego. The UCSD Press, La Jolla, California, 1993, pp 153-180.
7. UC San Diego Health: About Us – Awards and Achievements, https://health.ucsd.edu/about/pages/awards-achievements.aspx

8. Campaign to Raise $2.3M Toward Construction of Cancer Center and Medical Library at UC San Diego Medical Center, February 28, 1978, University Communications & Public Relations Materials: News Releases. Special Collections & Archives, UC San Diego Library.

9. Proposed Cancer Center To Be Named The Theodore Gildred Cancer Center, February 15, 1979, University Communications & Public Relations Materials: News Releases. Special Collections & Archives, UC San Diego Library.

10. UCSD to Conduct Capital Gift Campaign Toward Construction of Major Cancer Center, January 16, 1978, University Communications & Public Relations Materials: News Releases. Special Collections & Archives, UC San Diego Library.

11. Robert Erra Appointed Director of Hospital and Clinics and Associate Vice Chancellor for Health Sciences, May 4, 1982, University Communications & Public Relations Materials: News Releases. Special Collections & Archives, UC San Diego Library.

12. Richard C. Atkinson, Remarks at the School of Medicine 50th Anniversary Symposium, May 2, 2018.

13. UC Regents Approve Satellite Medical Facility, July 15, 1988, University Communications & Public Relations Materials: News Releases. Special Collections & Archives, UC San Diego Library.

14. Satellite Medical Facility (Thornton Hospital), July 13, 1988, University Communications & Public Relations Materials: News Releases. Special Collections & Archives, UC San Diego Library.

15. Architectural Designs for Satellite Medical Facility Approved, July 15, 1988, University Communications & Public Relations Materials: News Releases. Special Collections & Archives, UC San Diego Library.

16. UCSD's Shiley Eye Center Opening Gala Set for April 13, 1991, University Communications & Public Relations Materials: News Releases. Special Collections & Archives, UC San Diego Library.

17. Sumiyo Kastelic Retirement, Office of the Vice Chancellor for Health Sciences Communication, July 17, 2002.

18. UCSD Cancer Center Achieves Prestigious National Status, August 1, 2001, University Communications & Public Relations Materials: News Releases. Special Collections & Archives, UC San Diego Library.

19. John and Rebecca Moores Commit $20 Million Towards Planned UCSD Cancer Center Facility, May 4, 2000, University Communications & Public Relations Materials: News Releases. Special Collections & Archives, UC San Diego Library.

20. UCSD Names New Medical Center CEO, January 23, 2003, University Communications & Public Relations Materials: News Releases. Special Collections & Archives, UC San Diego Library.

21. UCSD Planning New Cardiovascular Center, Thornton Hospital Expansion, May 20, 2004, University Communications & Public Relations Materials: News Releases. Special Collections & Archives, UC San Diego Library.

22. Dedication Ceremony Marks Opening of New Moores UCSD Cancer Center Building, April 8, 2005, University Communications & Public Relations Materials: News Releases. Special Collections & Archives, UC San Diego Library.

23. UC San Diego Medical Center Breaks Ground for the Sulpizio Family Cardiovascular Center on September 27, September 26, 2007, University Communications & Public Relations Materials: News Releases. Special Collections & Archives, UC San Diego Library.

24. Regents Approve Plan for New UCSD Inpatient Bed Tower, May 28, 2007, University Communications & Public Relations Materials: News Releases. Special Collections & Archives, UC San Diego Library.

25. New CEO Named at UCSD Medical Center, November 19, 2009, University Communications & Public Relations Materials: News Releases. Special Collections & Archives, UC San Diego Library.

26. $52M NIH Grant Advances Clinical and Translational Research at UC San Diego, April 18, 2015, University Communications & Public Relations Materials: News Releases. Special Collections & Archives, UC San Diego Library.

27. UC Board of Regents Gives Approval for New Clinical and Translational Research Institute Building on UC San Diego's La Jolla Campus, November 19, 2010, University Communications & Public Relations Materials: News Releases. Special Collections & Archives, UC San Diego Library.

28. UC San Diego Health System Receives $75 Million Gift to Build New Medical Center, April 1, 2010, University Communications & Public Relations Materials: News Releases. Special Collections & Archives, UC San Diego Library.

29. 2010 Construction Projects at UC San Diego Total $568 million, January 31, 2010, University Communications & Public Relations Materials: News Releases. Special Collections & Archives, UC San Diego Library.

30. Altman Clinical and Translational Research Building Makes Its Debut, March 10, 2016, University Communications & Public Relations Materials: News Releases. Special Collections & Archives, UC San Diego Library.

31. Paul S. Viviano Named New CEO of UC San Diego Health System, May 1, 2012, University Communications & Public Relations Materials: News Releases. Special Collections & Archives, UC San Diego Library.

32. Looking Back and Ahead, Shiley's Vision Remains Clear, February 26, 2015, University Communications & Public Relations Materials: News Releases. Special Collections & Archives, UC San Diego Library.

33. Patty Maysent Named CEO of UC San Diego Health, January 21, 2016, University Communications & Public Relations Materials: News Releases. Special Collections & Archives, UC San Diego Library.

34. $52M NIH Grant Advances Clinical and Translational Research at UC San Diego, April 18, 2015, University Communications & Public Relations Materials: News Releases. Special Collections & Archives, UC San Diego Library.

35. UC San Diego Health to Open Jacobs Medical Center, November 20, 2016, November 17, 2016, University Communications & Public Relations Materials: News Releases. Special Collections & Archives, UC San Diego Library.

36. Koman Family Outpatient Pavilion Opens at UC San Diego Health on March 12, March 5, 2018, http://ucsdnews.ucsd.edu/pressrelease/koman_family_outpatient_pavilion_opens_at_uc_san_dieso_health_on_March_12

37. UC San Diego Center for Novel Therapeutics, April 2016 (Pre-Construction Plans), http://physicalplanning.ucsd.edu/pdf/projectsheets/center%20for%20novel%20therapeutics.pdf

Chapter 7

Growth of the Medical School West Campus

While the clinical enterprise was growing on both the Hillcrest and east campuses, the educational and research missions were expanding on the west campus in La Jolla.

The Buildings

As previously described, the first building on the school of medicine La Jolla campus was the Basic Sciences Building (subsequently renamed the Biomedical Sciences Building), opened in 1968 at a cost of $15.5 million [1]. Amazingly, the school managed to function with only one academic structure for ten years until the Medical Teaching Facility was opened in 1978 [Gary Matthews, personal communication, March 17, 2017]. The latter facility was a misnomer since, while it contained some classrooms, it housed mostly offices and laboratories for faculty.

Almost another ten years passed before the advent of a third building on the west campus: the Center for Molecular Genetics (later renamed the Center for Neural Circuits and Behavior) opened in 1987 at a cost of $7.6 million. This three-story building had 21,400 asf of laboratory space and 5,000 asf for an executive office wing. It was funded by the W.M. Keck Foundation as well as the University of California. The Howard Hughes Medical Institute contributed toward funding the facility's conference and meeting rooms. The building would house seven molecular genetics laboratories and a computer complex. Fifty faculty would be members of the center [2].

Following the recruitment of George Palade, M.D. as the school of medicine's first dean for scientific affairs, the Cellular and Molecular Medicine West building opened in 1990 [Gary

Matthews, personal communication, March 17, 2017]. This building (renamed the George Palade Laboratories for Cellular and Molecular Medicine in 2004) provided much needed research space for both new recruitments and individuals whose space in the Biomedical Sciences Building was inadequate.

In 1991 the Sam and Rose Stein Clinical Research Building, described by some as looking like an "inverted camera lens," opened [3]. The building would house the Institute for Research on Aging, a UC San Diego Organized Research Unit. A few years later, in 1995, Cellular and Molecular Medicine East, the "mirror image" of Cellular and Molecular Medicine West opened [Gary Matthews, personal communication, March 17, 2017; 4]. This new building's occupants would include the Ludwig Institute for Cancer Research [David N. Bailey, personal recollections and research].

The Keck Magnetic Resonance Imaging Facility, which opened in 2002, housed the Center for Functional Magnetic Resonance Imaging, a core research facility [5], while in 2004, the 140,000 asf, four-story Leichtag Family Foundation Biomedical Research Facility opened its doors. The foundation supported research on childhood diseases and provided a $12 million naming gift. Additional support was derived through the Garamendi mechanism, a State of California initiative which permitted use of National Institutes of Health (NIH) indirect cost recovery to pay for construction of buildings containing new NIH-funded research [3, 6]. The Howard Hughes Medical Institute (HHMI) also provided $10 million of support toward construction of the fourth floor of the building to house HHMI investigators [David N. Bailey, personal recollections and research].

Also, in 2004, a $17.7 million renovation and expansion of the biomedical library was launched in response to repeated recommendations of the Liaison Committee on Medical Education during onsite surveys. The original library, built in 1969 to serve only 800 users, had 27,764 asf. The expansion added 23,334 asf to serve more than 4,000 users [David N. Bailey, personal recollections and research; 7].

Although not a part of the school of medicine, in 2006 the Pharmaceutical Sciences Building was opened as the home of the Skaggs School of Pharmacy and Pharmaceutical Sciences, which had been established in 2002. This $45 million building included 45,000 square feet of wet laboratory and informatics space, 14,000 square feet of classroom space, and a 14,500 square foot education center for the health sciences [8].

A lull in west campus construction then occurred until 2010 when the nine-story, $67 million Rita Atkinson Residences, the first housing for health sciences professional and graduate students, opened. This structure had 225 two-bedroom apartment units and was named for Rita Atkinson, the wife of former University of California President and UC San Diego Chancellor Richard Atkinson, in recognition of her financial support for the facility [David N. Bailey, personal recollections and research; 9].

In 2011 the Sanford Consortium for Regenerative Medicine, a $127 million facility, was opened on UC San Diego land with funding provided by the State of California stem cell initiative and philanthropy, the lead donor being T. Denny Sanford. The 501c3 consortium members were UC San Diego, The Scripps Research Institute, The Salk Institute, The Sanford Burnham Prebys Medical Discovery Institute, and The La Jolla Institute for Allergy and

Immunology [David N. Bailey, personal recollections and research; 5]. This consortium provided a solution to the federal mandate that stem-cell projects could not be conducted with federal money and could not even be intermingled with federally sponsored projects [David N. Bailey, personal recollections and research]. Although technically not on the west campus of the school of medicine, this building was considered to be a vital part of the academic structure of the school.

The most exciting education building in the history of the school of medicine, the Medical Education and Telemedicine Building, was opened in the fall of 2011. This $70 million building was funded by $35 million in state funds via a proposition for telemedicine with debt funding and philanthropy for the remainder. The building contains 60,000 asf including telemedicine space, a 9,000 asf clinical skills and simulation center, 18 examination rooms, and simulated hospital room, intensive care unit, and emergency room. There is also a 6,800 asf medical and procedures teaching laboratory with 22 stations, classrooms, learning communities, and a computer-based testing facility. The basement of the building contains the Center for the Future of Surgery, equipped with two operating rooms containing state-of-the-art surgical equipment and laparoscopic instrumentation [4, 9, 10]. The impact of this facility on medical education and training was as transformational as that of the Jacobs Medical Center was on the clinical mission of the school! In December 2017 the building was named the T. Denny Sanford Medical Education and Telemedicine Center in recognition of the generosity and influential role of Denny Sanford in sparking research and collaboration across the health sciences [11].

The $36 million three-story, 42,000 gsf Centralized Research Support Facility, opened in 2013, houses a central equipment sanitation center, the UC San Diego Animal Care Program, and administrative offices. Centralization of services saved the campus untold dollars through improved efficiency. Of the funding for construction, $14 million came from the National Institutes of Health [Gary Matthews, personal communication, March 17, 2017; 12].

In 2013 J. Craig Venter, who, along with Francis Collins, was credited with first sequencing the human genome, expanded the J. Craig Venter Institute by constructing a building in La Jolla on UC San Diego property. Like the Sanford Consortium for Regenerative Medicine, this was not physically located on the West Campus nor under the authority of UC San Diego, but many of its employees had joint appointments in the UC San Diego School of Medicine, and it has enriched the academic milieu of the school [David N. Bailey, personal recollections and research; 3].

Finally, in 2014, the $113 million, 196,000 asf Health Sciences Biomedical Research Facility II opened its doors with Leadership in Energy and Environmental Design (LEED) platinum certification (the highest designation for green design and operation). The building was only the second UC San Diego building to receive platinum certification. This facility brought together interdisciplinary groups working in thematic areas (e.g., immunology, glycobiology, gastrointestinal diseases, cardiovascular diseases, infectious diseases) [David N. Bailey, personal recollections and research; 13]. The building capitalized on lessons learned from construction of prior research buildings in the school of medicine.

The Organized Research Units Based in the School of Medicine

In the University of California system an organized research unit (ORU) is an academic unit that provides a supportive infrastructure for interdisciplinary research complementary to the academic goals of formal departments. An ORU facilitates research and research collaborations; disseminates research results through research conferences, meetings, and other activities; strengthens graduate and undergraduate education by providing students with training opportunities and access to facilities; seeks extramural funding; and carries out university and public service programs related to the unit's research expertise. An ORU may not offer formal courses for credit to university students or to the public unless approved by the university to do so. Each ORU has a commitment of space and funding. Establishment and continuation of ORUs after formal review follow established university and campus policies [David N. Bailey, personal recollections and research; 14].

Although there are numerous ORUs at UC San Diego, the UC San Diego School of Medicine is enriched by having eight based in the school. These are described below in chronological order of establishment.

Cancer Center (1979)

The first organized research unit was the Cancer Center, established in 1979, although it had existed since 1978 as a non-ORU center. The directors and their years of appointment were John Mendelsohn, M.D. (1979), Mark Green, M.D. (1985), William Hryniuk, M.D. (1992), David Tarin, M.D. (1997), Dennis Carson, M.D. (2003), and Scott Lippmann (2012), all professors of medicine except for David Tarin, who was professor of pathology [David N. Bailey, personal recollections and research]. The Cancer Center ceased to operate as an organized research unit in 2017.

Stein Institute for Research on Aging (1983)

This was the second ORU at UC San Diego. Although originally the institute's focus was on Alzheimer's disease, it has broadened to include mechanisms involved in the aging process and chronic diseases of the elderly. The founding director was J. Edwin Seegmiller, M.D., professor of medicine. Dennis Carson, M.D., professor of medicine, assumed the directorship in 1990, and Dilip Jeste, M.D., professor of psychiatry, became director in 2004 [4, 15].

AIDS Research Institute (1996)

The AIDS Research Institute was established in 1996 to coordinate the diverse Acquired Immunodeficiency Syndrome (AIDS) research and clinical activities of UCSD [16]. The founding and still current director is Douglas Richman, M.D., professor of pathology.

Center for Research in Biological Systems (1996)

Created in 1996, this ORU provides an integrative framework to facilitate multiscale studies of biological systems. The founding and current director is Mark Ellisman, Ph.D., professor of neurosciences [David N. Bailey, personal recollections and research; 17].

Glycobiology Research and Training Center (1999)

This ORU, established in 1999, is a virtual center without walls whose mission is to facilitate and enhance glycobiology research and training. The founding and still current director is Ajit Varki, M.D., professor of medicine [18].

Altman Clinical and Translational Research Institute (2004)

Originally called the Clinical Investigation Institute, the Clinical and Translational Research Institute was founded in 2004 with Gary Firestein, M.D., professor of medicine and dean for translational research, as founding and still current director. In 2011 the institute received a naming gift from Steve and Lisa Altman [David N. Bailey, personal recollections and research; 3, 19].

Center for Academic Research and Training in Anthropogeny (CARTA) (2008)

This virtual ORU was established in 2008 to promote transdisciplinary research into human origins, drawing on methods from traditional disciplines spanning the social, biomedical, biological, computational, and the engineering, physical and chemical sciences as well as the humanities. The founding and still current director is Ajit Varki, M.D., professor of medicine [David N. Bailey, personal recollections and research; 20].

Institute for Genomic Medicine (2009)

This institute, launched in 2009, coalesces UC San Diego's strengths in basic science, disease biology, pharmacology, engineering, clinical research, and computer science to accelerate investigation and translation in genetics and genomic medicine. The founding director was Kang Zhang, M.D., Ph.D., professor of ophthalmology. The current director is Kelly Frazer, Ph.D., professor of pediatrics, appointed in 2013 [21].

Affiliated Research Institutes Based on the School of Medicine Campus

In 1991, shortly after appointment of George Palade, M.D. as the school of medicine founding dean for scientific affairs, UC San Diego signed an affiliation agreement with the Ludwig Institute for Cancer Research to create a cancer research collaboration. Ludwig investigators were subsequently appointed as UC San Diego ladder-rank faculty. Space in the Cellular and Molecular Medicine East building was leased by the institute. The founding director of the institute was Webster Cavenee, Ph.D., professor of medicine. In 2015 Richard Kolodner, Ph.D., professor of cellular and molecular medicine, became director [David N. Bailey, personal recollections and research; 22].

In 1996, again during George Palade's tenure, the Howard Hughes Medical Institute established an affiliation agreement with UC San Diego, similar to that of the Ludwig Institute, with investigators being appointed as UC San Diego ladder-rank faculty and research space being leased from the university [3].

In 2015 the La Jolla Institute for Allergy & Immunology, located in UC San Diego research science park on the east campus, signed an affiliation agreement with UC San Diego, in which institute members would become adjunct faculty in the school of medicine [23]. Although not on the west campus this institute contributes significantly to the research mission of the school and thus is included in this chapter.

Finally, the east and west campuses are being linked by a bridge across Interstate 5. In a sense this bridge also symbolizes a link between the research/education and the clinical missions of the school. As with the clinical enterprise, the academic enterprise had grown just as aggressively, propelling UC San Diego School of Medicine to international prominence.

References

1. N.A. Anderson. An Improbable Venture: A History of the University of California, San Diego. The UCSD Press, La Jolla, California, 1993, pp. 153-180.
2. Center for Molecular Genetics Building Opens, May 4, 1987, University Communications & Public Relations Materials: News Releases. Special Collections & Archives, UC San Diego Library.
3. UC San Diego Health: About Us – Awards and Achievements, https://health.ucsd.edu/about/pages/awards-achievements.aspx
4. UC San Diego Health: About Us – Our History, https://health.ucsd.edu/about/pages/history.aspx
5. UC San Diego School of Medicine Center for Functional MRI, https://cfmriweb.ucsd.edu/
6. L. Franz: UCSD Dedicates Leichtag Biomedical Research Building, April 27, 2004, http://ucsdnews.ucsd.edu/archive/newsrel/health/04_27_Leichtag.asp
7. Expansion and Renovation of UCSD's Biomedical Library Slated to Begin with July 20 Groundbreaking Ceremony, July 8, 2004, University Communications & Public Relations Materials: News Releases. Special Collections & Archives, UC San Diego Library.
8. UCSD Skaggs School of Pharmacy & Pharmaceutical Sciences – Second Public School of Pharmacy in CA – Officially Opens Its Doors, April 27, 2006, University Communications & Public Relations Materials: News Releases. Special Collections & Archives, UC San Diego Library.
9. 2010 Construction Projects at UC San Diego Total $568 Million, January 13, 2010, University Communications & Public Relations Materials: News Releases. Special Collections & Archives, UC San Diego Library.
10. UC San Diego School of Medicine to Build an Innovative Hub of Learning for the 21st Century, November 23, 2009, University Communications & Public Relations Materials: News Releases. Special Collections & Archives, UC San Diego Library.
11. Giving Hope for a Better Future, December 13, 2017, https://chancellor.ucsd.edu/chancellor-khosla/blog/giving-hope-for-a-better-future
12. Tradeline Inc., Centralized Research Facility Reaping Significant Benefits, March 1, 2017, https://www.tradelineinc.com/reports/2017-2/centralized-research-support-facility-reaping-significant-benefits
13. S. LaFee: UC San Diego Health, Biomedical Research Facility II Receives LEED Platinum Certification, December 22, 2015, https://health.ucsd.edu/news/releases/Pages/2015-12-22-Biomedical-Research-Facility-II-Receives-LEED-Platinum-Certification.aspx
14. University of California Administrative Policies and Procedures Concerning Organized Research Units, December 7, 1999, http://policy.ucop.edu/doc/2500488/ORU

15. UCSD Medical School Plans Institute of Aging, October 7, 1985, University Communications & Public Relations Materials: News Releases. Special Collections & Archives, UC San Diego Library.
16. UC San Diego AIDS Research Institute, https://healthsciences.ucsd.edu/research/pages/arc.aspx
17. UC San Diego Center for Research in Biological Systems, http://crbs.ucsd.edu/about/mission
18. UC San Diego Glycobiology Research and Training Center, https://healthsciences.ucsd.edu/research/pages/grtc.aspx
19. UCSD Announces Appointment of Clinical Investigation Institute Director, September 8, 2003, University Communications & Public Relations. Materials: News Releases. Special Collections & Archives, UC San Diego Library
20. UC San Diego Center for Academic Research and Training in Anthropogeny (CARTA), https://carta.anthropogeny.org/about/carta
21. Campus Notice, Office of the Vice Chancellor Health Sciences/Dean. School of Medicine, June 19, 2009: Institute for Genomic Medicine.
22. UC San Diego Ludwig Institute for Cancer Research at UCSD, https://healthsciences.ucsd.edu/pages/ludwig-institute-for-cancer-research-(LICR).aspx
23. G. Robbins: Institute Spurns USC, Chooses UC San Diego, *San Diego Union-Tribune*, July 25, 2015.

Chapter 8

Faculty Academic Series

By its very nature academic medicine is difficult at best as individuals struggle to balance the missions of research, teaching, and service (clinical service, university service, and public service). Most schools of medicine now have both clinician-educator and clinician-scientist academic series to recognize the fact that faculty may have different emphases in their careers. Assuring that faculty are placed into the proper academic series is of paramount importance in assuring their success. Since academic series define and shape faculty culture, this chapter is included in this book.

While the academic appointment, merit advancement, and promotion process is complicated in most places, the University of California (UC) system is very byzantine, to say the least. This will be readily attested to by the many external reviewers who are asked repeatedly to write letters of evaluation for candidates under review. The UC system has six steps of assistant professor, five steps of associate professor, nine steps of full professor, and an unlimited number of "above scale" ("distinguished professor") advancements. Each step is a defined period of time so that every faculty member (including all tenured faculty) are reviewed at regular time intervals. For those whose files do not show sufficient progress to warrant advancement, there is even a "no change" merit review. Assistant professors undergo a formal "fourth-year appraisal" as they enter the fourth year of appointment. This appraisal, proposed by the department, and then overseen by a separate body of reviewers, judges performance to be "favorable," "favorable with reservations," "problematic," and "unfavorable" for promotion to associate rank two to four years hence if the candidate continues on the same trajectory.

Assistant-rank faculty can remain for only eight years, and then must be terminated if they do not advance to associate rank. All faculty, except for tenured faculty, have term appointments which must be renewed for continuation at fixed time intervals. "Career" reviews, using evaluations from external referees along with the teaching, research, and service dossiers, occur on promotion to associate rank, to professor rank, and to "above scale" ("distinguished professor") rank. A special review also occurs for advancement to professor, step VI (the so-called "barrier" step) [David N. Bailey, personal recollections and research].

The University of California has five professorial series, each of which is discussed below, and each of which is currently used for the 1,463 school of medicine faculty that existed in 2016. Three of these series (ladder-rank, in residence, and clinical X) convey Academic Senate membership while two (adjunct and health sciences clinical series) do not. The Academic Senate is the mechanism for faculty to participate in shared governance with University administration. Members can sit on standing committees of the Academic Senate, can vote on appointments and promotions of other Senate members of the same or lower rank in their department, and can apply for Senate travel awards and research grants among other perquisites. Furthermore, appointments must be at 100% time while non-Senate faculty can have fractional, reduced-time employment depending upon funding availability. The title of "emeritus" professor is given automatically to Senate members upon their retirement while such title is available only by exception for non-Senate members on retirement after at least ten years of service and attainment of the rank of full professor [1; David N. Bailey, personal recollections and research].

Ladder-Rank Series

The ladder-rank series is the original academic series in the University of California. Used predominantly by general campus faculty, this series requires that at least half of the base ("X" component) salary be supported by a state-funded FTE (line). This is the only series that grants tenure, which is awarded on promotion to associate rank. The number of FTEs assigned to each school was originally determined by formula based on the number of students. Older schools of medicine such as those at UC Los Angeles and UC San Francisco were granted many more FTEs than younger ones like UC San Diego, which in 2016 had grown to only 250 FTEs for its 1,463 faculty [David N. Bailey, personal recollections and research; Andrew L. Ries, personal communication, June 20, 2017]!

The ladder-rank series emphasizes research with excellence in teaching and service (both University and public service). Being an Academic Senate series, appointments must be 100% time, and the campus Committee on Academic Personnel is the final arbiter for academic advancements. Of interest, all founding faculty (chapter 4) were appointed in the ladder-rank series except for two, who were appointed in the In Residence series (see description below). In those days, research funding from the National Institutes of Health was relatively easy to acquire, research was less expensive, and single-investigator projects were the norm, thereby making it easier for clinical faculty to conduct research programs while being very active clinically and educationally. Furthermore, class sizes were smaller, classroom lectures were the norm, patient population was smaller, and clinical reimbursements were better. Perhaps, just as importantly, administrative "beaurocracy" (particularly in the clinical arena) was much less [David N. Bailey, personal recollections and research].

As the demands of patient practice and education grew and as the support for research shrank, appointments in other academic series grew. As of today, appointments in the ladder-rank series are reserved largely for basic scientists whose research is believed to be transformational. In 2016, the school of medicine had only 317 faculty (21.7% of total) in this series [Andrew L. Ries, personal communication, June 20, 2017].

In Residence Series

Requirements for appointment and advancement in the in residence series are the same as that for the ladder-rank series. However, funding must come from sources other than the state (e.g., clinical income, research grant support). Most faculty in this series fund salaries from grant income since clinical activity usually leaves insufficient time for research. Being an Academic Senate series, appointments must be 100% time, which frequently is challenging since salary support must be self-generated, and, as with the ladder-rank series, academic advancements are overseen by the campus Committee on Academic Personnel. Thus, not surprisingly, this series has the smallest number of faculty in the school of medicine - in 2016, 104 faculty (7.1%) [1; David N. Bailey, personal recollections and research; Andrew L. Ries, personal communication, June 20, 2017].

Adjunct Series

The adjunct series is a very flexible series with advancement being based on achievements in research and teaching or research and clinical service depending upon the distribution of effort, which is generally more specialized than that in either the ladder-rank or in residence series. Since this is not an Academic Senate series, appointments can be fractional, based upon availability of funding.   Despite not being an Academic Senate series, academic advancements are overseen by the campus Committee on Academic Personnel since research and university service are requirements for this series. As with the in residence series, few school of medicine faculty are in this track – in 2016, 168 faculty (11.5%) [1; David N. Bailey, personal recollections and research; Andrew L. Ries, personal communication, June 20, 2017].

Health Sciences Clinical Series

The health sciences clinical series exists only in the health sciences and is intended for faculty whose primary responsibilities are in clinical work and teaching. Thus the adjunct series (which requires research) is not appropriate for these individuals. That said, scholarly activity of some type (e.g., case reports, reviews, practice guidelines) is required. Since this is not an Academic Senate series, appointments can be less than 100%, and reappointments occur annually up to professor, step VI, after which reappointments are for the duration of the step. Salaries are usually supported by clinical income. Academic advancements are reviewed internally by the School of Medicine Committee on Academic Personnel instead of by campus reviewers. Since the series emphasizes clinical work with teaching often occurring concurrently, this series is the largest in the school of medicine – in 2016, 749 faculty (51.2%) [1; David N. Bailey, personal recollections and research; Andrew L. Ries, personal communication, June 20, 2017].

Clinical X Series

This is the newest academic track, created in 1987 for outstanding clinician teachers in response to faculty concerns that clinicians were denied the benefits of Academic Senate membership (outlined above). Due to concerns by the Academic Senate that clinicians might "override" votes of non-clinical Academic Senate faculty, a percent cap based on number of Senate faculty in each department was initially placed on the number of faculty allowed in this series. Over time the cap has been largely ignored. The "X" in the clinical X series denotes a particular discipline (e.g., medicine, pediatrics) (e.g., professor of clinical medicine, professor of clinical pediatrics). Like the health sciences clinical series, this track is reserved for health sciences faculty who excel in teaching and clinical work. However, unlike the health sciences clinical series, faculty are expected to show significant creative activity and generally to carry a heavier load of teaching and clinical work than ladder-rank and in residence faculty. Since this is an Academic Senate series, appointments must be 100% time, and salaries are usually supported significantly by clinical income. Academic advancement is overseen by the campus Committee on Academic personnel although the school of medicine Committee on Academic Personnel provides preliminary input. In 2016 there were 125 faculty (8.5%) in this series, making it next to the smallest series in the school [1; David N. Bailey, personal recollections and research; Andrew L. Ries, personal communication, June 20, 2017].

The health sciences clinical and clinical X series together account for 59.7% of medical school faculty [Andrew L. Ries, personal communication, June 20, 2017] and are the most rapidly growing series. All tracks (except for clinical X, initiated in 1987) were available from the founding of the school. Despite the growing number of clinical faculty, additional faculty are needed to provide clinical teaching, and, for this reason, several thousand voluntary clinical faculty outside the University have been added as well as non-salaried clinical faculty (i.e., University employees who are not employed by the school itself but who desire to teach without compensation). These appointments are handled internally within the school. Non-salaried adjunct faculty appointments are used for research faculty outside the university (e.g., the adjacent research institutes) who provide largely non-clinical teaching to medical and graduate students. These appointments are reviewed and renewed at regular intervals with oversight by the campus Committee on Academic Personnel. A fulltime research series (e.g., research pathologist, research microbiologist) and a lecturer series are also available but, since these are not considered professorial series, a discussion of them is not included here [David N. Bailey, personal recollections and research].

Since the founding of the school. use of the academic series has evolved considerably. As previously noted, at this time the ladder-rank series is used primarily for basic scientists whose research is transformative. The role of the clinical X series has, in this author's view, replaced that of the ladder-rank series in the earlier days with focus on applied and translational research while the health sciences clinical series continues to be used mostly for clinicians who provide teaching along with their service as well as some scholarly and creative activity. With the advent of the two clinical series, the adjunct series has become one primarily for faculty who are research-focused and who provide some teaching [David N. Bailey, personal recollections and research].

Although the variety of academic series has permitted faculty to find an appropriate niche for themselves, it has also created a perception of classes of "citizenship," with "gold-card" membership being reserved for Academic Senate members (ladder-rank, in residence, clinical X), who enjoy the benefits outlined above, and "platinum-card" membership reserved for the fortunate few who are given FTEs (ladder-rank faculty who can earn tenure and who do not have to be reappointed). Adjunct and health sciences clinical faculty are not Academic Senate members.

References

1. Overview of the Faculty Series, March 8, 2004, https://healthsciences.ucsd.edu/vchs/faculty-academics/faculty-council/documents/faculty-series030804.pdf

Chapter 9

The "Enablers"

In almost every medical school there are staff whose creativity, hard work, many years of service, and dedication help to create the vital force or "life blood" of the school. These often "unsung heroes" make things happen by working behind the scenes.   While UC San Diego School of Medicine has been fortunate to have had a number of talented people, this chapter will focus on a few special "enablers" in chronological order of their appointments.

Roger Meyer, Associate Dean for Administration (1971 – 2002) [Roger Meyer, personal communication, May 27, 2017; David N. Bailey, personal recollections and research]

Roger Meyer received his Bachelor of Science degree in psychology and mathematics from Yankton College (Yankton, South Dakota) and his Master of Science degree in industrial management from the University of North Dakota. After seven years of service as an officer in the United States Air Force, Roger joined the UC San Diego School of Medicine dean's office as an operations officer in 1971. In 1974, under Dean Moxley, he was appointed Assistant Dean for Administration, and in 1981 he was promoted to Associate Dean for Administration and Associate Vice Chancellor for Health Sciences Administration.

During Mr. Meyer's 31 years of service to the dean's office he oversaw the finances of the school of medicine (about $400 million of activity per year in his final years) and was the person responsible for school budgets and resources to support mission needs. He also developed the school's affirmative action programs; managed the school's administrative and infrastructure information technology; oversaw the schools' contracts, grants, and legal agreements (at least $300 million annually); served as the senior non-academic advisor to the dean and department chairs on organizational structure and direction; and was the primary liaison for the school to major campus support offices. On the national level Roger served as chairperson to the Association of American Medical Colleges (AAMC) Group on Business Affairs.

Throughout his service to the many medical school deans the phrase "give it to Roger, and he will handle it" was common. Roger Meyer was indeed the "go-to," "make it happen" person.

Ruth Covell, M.D., Associate Dean for Planning and Policy (1976 – 2011) [David N. Bailey, personal recollections and research; Ruth M. Covell, personal communication, June 27, 2017]

When she was only two years old, Ruth Covell told her mother that she wanted to be a pediatrician. She persisted in pursuing her dream although she ended up training in internal medicine instead of pediatrics. Having received her Bachelor of Arts degree from Stanford, where she was elected to Phi Beta Kappa honorary, she received her Doctor of Medicine degree from the University of Chicago, where she was elected to Alpha Omega Alpha medical honorary. Following a residency in internal medicine at the University of Chicago, she then migrated into medical officer positions in the United States Public Health Service, focusing on planning and evaluation. Prior to arriving at UC San Diego School of Medicine she was senior medical advisor in the Office of the Director of Health Standards and Quality Bureau of the Health Care Financing Administration. In 1976 Ruth Covell was appointed assistant dean for policy and planning under Dean John Moxley. In 1981 she became associate dean, and in 1985 she also became Director of the UC San Diego Academic Geriatric Resource Center. She retired from UC San Diego in 2011.

Over her 35 years of service in the UC San Diego School of Medicine dean's office, Ruth oversaw many specialized projects that were transformational for the school. These projects included, but were not limited to, securing extramural funding for the Clinical Teaching Facility, the Medical Teaching Facility, the fourth floor of the Stein Clinical Research Building, the first floor of the Cellular and Molecular Medicine West building, and the Keck Functional Magnetic Resonance Imaging Center. She also obtained extramural funding to help launch the original medical school tutorial program as well as funding for the UC San Diego Academic Geriatric Resource Center and the nurse practitioner program. Additionally, Ruth played a significant role in obtaining approval for construction of the John M and Sally B Thornton Hospital and in establishment of the Skaggs School of Pharmacy and Pharmaceutical Sciences.

Aside from these accomplishments she played a major role in the development of the master plans for the school of medicine and served on the Campus Community Planning Committee, chairing it every third year. She led the school's preparations for Liaison Committee on Medical Education (LCME) reaccreditation for many years. As Clinical Professor of Family Medicine and Public Health, she established the first course in Health Care System in the country when she arrived at UC San Diego. She also helped to found the San Ysidro Health Centers, which operates integrated health centers across south San Diego, currently serving more than 450,000 underserved patients per year. Finally she was a founder of Community Health Improvement Partners (CHIP) in 1995, a group to assess and address community health needs.

Dr. Covell's honors include the University of Chicago Division of Medicine and Biological Sciences Distinguished Service Award, the UC San Diego Emeriti Association Dickson Award for her continued service to the university and for her mentoring of students after retirement, and the CHIP Lifetime Achievement Award. She was also honored by the San Diego City Council with the declaration of June 30, 2013, to be "Dr. Ruth Covell Day."

Lourdes Felix, Executive Assistant to the Vice Chancellor for Health Sciences and Dean of the School of Medicine (1986 – 2012) [David N. Bailey, personal recollections and research; Lourdes Felix, personal communication, May 30, 2017]

Lourdes ("Lou") Felix graduated from UC San Diego with a Bachelor of Arts degree in Latin American and English Literature and spent her entire career at UC San Diego, initially serving as an administrative assistant in the departments of surgery and biology before becoming an administrative assistant in the school of medicine dean's office. In 1986, she was appointed Executive Assistant to Vice Chancellor and Dean Petersdorf and subsequently served in that role to vice chancellor and dean Akeson (interim), Burrow, Alksne, Bailey (interim twice), Holmes, and Brenner. She retired in 2012. Her numerous recognitions included the UC San Diego Diversity Award, the UC San Diego Cross Cultural Center Recognition Award, and the UC San Diego Top-Ten Employee of the Year Award, among others.

The word around the school was that "Lou trained seven deans"! Although that may seem like a stretch, in reality it was true. Ms. Felix's guidance and knowledge of the UC system, coupled with her calm demeanor and sense of humor, made the lives of each vice chancellor/dean better and contributed to their success. She also was the ever pleasant, charming "face" of the vice chancellor/dean's office. More than once, departing vice chancellors/deans lamented that they would miss Lou more than anyone else! Just as importantly, Lou was a mentor to underrepresented students and staff, helping them to advance in their education and training. A number of UC San Diego senior staff today express their gratitude to Lou Felix for their careers.

Chapter 10[*]

Secrets to Success

Within fifty years of admitting its first medical students the UC San Diego School of Medicine not only caught the wave but also continues to ride it. How did this happen? Why did this young institution flourish while others, founded at about the same time, floundered?

One very astute senior faculty member noted that "The rapid ascendance and tremendous success of the UC San Diego School of Medicine resulted from a confluence of strategic decisions made by the <u>right people</u> with the <u>right vision</u> in the <u>right place</u> at the <u>right time</u>."

These strategic decisions included an initial <u>focus on basic science</u>, which permeated the fabric of the school from its creation, leaving a long-lasting imprint on its culture. The <u>location of the school</u> on the campus of a research-intensive university with illustrious neighboring research institutes nurtured this decision. Additionally, aside from the ideal climate of San Diego, the location was <u>geographically buffered</u> in all directions from other competing schools. With essentially <u>a blank canvas</u>, there was tremendous opportunity to create a new model for a school of medicine, unfettered by tradition that often handicaps more established schools. Furthermore, in the culture of the University of California system, <u>governance was bottom up and not top down,</u> allowing faculty to be left alone to develop their research programs.

Although the initial focus of the school was on basic science, which was driven in part by the need to have faculty to teach the preclinical curriculum, the clinical and translational medicine followed, albeit at a slower pace, due largely to the lack of an adequate clinical environment in which to teach in the early years. As expansion of the clinical enterprise occurred, clinical and translational medicine grew, culminating with the development of a new medical center on the east campus.

The timing for creation of the school was also ideal, given the veritable explosion of scientific advancements in molecular biology coupled with the large investment in research from the National Institutes of Health (NIH) and other agencies. A "bolus" of world-renowned, pioneering, entrepreneurial faculty were recruited as founding department chairs from the NIH and other institutions with an emphasis on individuals who thought "out of the box" and who were not afraid to take risks. Subsequently, a few world-class leaders such as George Palade were added, and they served as "magnets," quickly drawing talent and resources, each of which had a multiplication effect.

The impact of visionary deans/vice chancellors coupled with unwavering support of enlightened campus chancellors, many of whom were basic scientists, further facilitated rapid growth and development of the school.

Despite its emphasis on basic science, the unique departmental model of the school, which embedded basic science in the clinical departments created a synergy between the two, allowing for evolution of only a few basic science departments over time (i.e., Pharmacology, Cellular and Molecular Medicine). Other disciplines such as physiology, immunology, microbiology, and biochemistry largely remain integrated within clinical departments today.

The innovative curriculum was non-departmental, allowing interdisciplinary input into courses instead of competition between department for teaching time. Grades were deemphasized from the beginning, and student independent study and research projects were encouraged from the outset.

All of these ingredients together resulted in a school characterized by relentless innovation, tremendous collaboration, and extensive outreach to the community. Although it is a cliché, "success breeds success," and the UC San Diego School of Medicine from the outset has been a success. Amazingly, the wave has not subsidized, and the ride continues!

*These reflections were informed by communications from John F. Alksne, Elizabeth Barrett-Connor, Marilyn G. Farquhar, Steven Garfin, Gordon Gill, Joan Heller-Brown, Roger Meyer, Thomas R. Moore, William Nyhan, Marshall J. Orloff, Andrew L. Ries, Palmer W. Taylor, and John West.

APPENDICES

Appendix A: Deans*

Joseph Stokes (1964 – 1966)

Robert Tschirgi (1967) (Interim)

Clifford Grobstein (1967 – 1973)

John Moxley (1973 – 1979)

Marvin Dunn (1979 – 1980) (Interim)

William Hollingsworth (1980 – 1981 (Interim)

Robert G. Petersdorf (1981 – 1986)

Wayne Akeson (1986 – 1988) (Interim)

Gerard N. Burrow (1988 – 1992)

John F. Alksne (1992 – 1999)

David N. Bailey (1999 – 2000) (Interim)

Edward W. Holmes (2000 – 2006)

David N. Bailey (2006 – 2007) (Interim)

David A. Brenner (2007 – present as vice chancellor; 2007 – 2018 as dean)

Steven Garfin (2018 – present) (Interim dean)

*Up through David A. Brenner, the deans were also vice chancellors for health sciences. Beginning in 2018 the position of vice chancellor and dean was bifurcated.

Appendix B: Chairs of Academic Departments

(Arranged in Alphabetical Order by Department)

Anesthesiology

1974 - Lawrence Saidman

1985 - Harvey Shapiro

1997 - John C. Drummond

2004 - Gerard Manecke (Interim)

2008 - Gerard Manecke

2018 – Ruth Waterman (Interim)

Cellular and Molecular Medicine

1999 - Marilyn G. Farquhar

2008 - Donald Cleveland

Dermatology

2015 - Richard Gallo

Emergency Medicine

2013 - Theodore Chan

Family Medicine and Public Health

1966 - Joseph Stokes III (Department of Preventive Medicine)

1974 - Doris Howell (Department of Community and Family Medicine)

1981 – Elizabeth Barrett-Connor (Interim)

1982 - Elizabeth Barrett-Connor

1997 - Robert Kaplan (Department of Family and Preventive Medicine) (Interim)

1999 - Robert Kaplan

2004 - Theodore Ganiats (Interim)

2011 - Bess Marcus (Department of Family Medicine and Public Health)

2017 – Cheryl Anderson (Interim)

Medicine

1968 - Eugene Braunwald

1972 - Nathan Zvaifler (Interim)

1973 - Helen M. Ranney

1986 - Stephen Wasserman (Interim)

1988 - Stephen Wasserman

2000 - Roger Spragg (Interim)

2002 - Kenneth Kaushansky

2010 - Wolfgang Dillmann (Interim)

2012 - Wolfgang Dillmann

Neurosciences

1965 - Robert Livingston

1970 - John O'Brien

1978 - Wigbert Wiederholt

1983 - Doris Trauner (Interim)

1984 - Robert Katzman

1993 - Leon Thal

2007 - Doris Trauner (Interim)

2009 - William Mobley

2016 - James Brewer (Interim)

2018 – James Brewer

Obstetrics, Gynecology, and Reproductive Sciences

1970 - Kenneth Ryan

1972 - Samuel Yen

1983 - Robert Resnik

1995 - Thomas Moore

2014 - Charles Nager (In 2018 - Department of Obstetrics, Gynecology, and Reproductive Sciences instead of Department of Reproductive Medicine)

Ophthalmology

1983 - Stuart Brown

2008 - Robert Weinreb

Orthopaedic Surgery

1991 - Wayne Akeson (Department of Orthopedics)

1996 - Steven Garfin (In 2003 – Department of Orthopaedic Surgery)

2018 – Reid Abrams (Interim)

Pathology

1967 - Averill Liebow

1975 - Colin M. Bloor (Interim)

1977 - Kurt Benirschke

1979 - Peter W. Lampert

1986 - David N. Bailey (Interim)

1988 - David N. Bailey

1999 - Henry C. Powell (Interim)

2000 - David N. Bailey

2001 - Henry C. Powell (Interim)

2004 - Steven L. Gonias

Pediatrics

1968 - Robert Hamburger

1969 - William Nyhan

1986 - Michael Kaback

1992 - Stanley Mendoza

2000 - Kenneth Lee Jones (Interim)

2005 - Gabriel Haddad

Pharmacology

1987 - Palmer W. Taylor

2002 - Joan Heller-Brown (Interim)

2005 - Joan Heller-Brown

Psychiatry

1969 - Arnold Mandell

1977 - Lewis Judd

2014 - Igor Grant

Radiation Medicine and Applied Sciences

2006 - A.J. Mundt

Radiology

1968 - Elliott Lasser

1977 - Robert N. Berk

1985 - George Leopold

2002 - William Bradley

2015 - Alexander Norbash

Surgery

1965 - Marshall J. Orloff

1983 - Abdul R. Moossa

2003 - David Hoyt (Interim)

2005 - Mark Talamini

2013 - Christopher Kane (Interim)

2015 - Bryan Clary

Urology

2017 - Christopher K. Kane

Appendix C: Directors of Organized Research Units

(Arranged in Alphabetical Order by Unit)

AIDS Research Institute

1996 -Douglas Richman

Altman Clinical and Translational Research Institute

2004 - Gary S. Firestein (2016 – Altman Clinical and Translational Research Institute)

Cancer Center (Discontinued as ORU in 2017)

1978 - John Mendelsohn

1985 - Mark Green

1992 - William Hryniuk

1997 - David Tarin

2003 - Dennis Carson (2005 – Rebecca and John Moores Cancer Center)

2012 - Scott Lippmann

Center for Academic Research and Training in Anthropogeny (CARTA)

2008 - Ajit Varki

Center for Research in Biological Systems

1996 - Mark Ellisman

Glycobiology Research and Training Center

1999 - Ajit Varki

Institute for Genomic Medicine

2009 - Kang Zhang

2013 - Kelly Frazer

Stein Institute for Research on Aging

1983 - J. Edwin Seegmiller

1990 - Dennis Carson

2004 - Dilip Jeste

Appendix D: Health System Chief Executive Officers

1966 - Richard A. Lockwood

1973 - Sheldon King

1981 - Vincent Wayne (Interim)

1982 - Robert Erra

1983 - Michael Stringer (Interim)

1984 - Michael Stringer

1997 - Sumiyo Kastelic

2002 - Richard Liekweg

2010 - Thomas Jackiewicz

2012 - Paul Viviano

2015 - Patty Maysent (Interim)

2016 - Patty Maysent

Appendix E: Clinical Practice Sites[*]

Medical Center-Based Sites:

UC San Diego Medical Center – Hillcrest, 200 West Arbor Drive, San Diego, California 92103

Medical Offices North, 200 West Arbor Drive, San Diego, California 92103

Jacobs Medical Center (including Thornton Pavilion), 9300 Campus Point Drive, La Jolla, California 92037

Perlman Medical Offices, 9350 Campus Point Drive, La Jolla, California 92037

Moores Cancer Center, 3855 Health Sciences Drive, La Jolla, California 92037

Sulpizio Cardiovascular Center, 9434 Medical Center Drive, La Jolla, California 92037

Shiley Eye Institute, 9415 Campus Point Drive, La Jolla, California 92037

Altman Clinical and Translational Research Institute, 9452 Medical Center Drive, La Jolla, California 92037

PET/CT Center (Radiation Oncology), 3960 Health Sciences Drive, La Jolla, California 92093

Outpatient Clinics:

Sites That Are Part of UC San Diego Health, La Jolla –

4510 and 4520 Executive Drive, San Diego, California 92121

8899 and 8929 University Center Lane, San Diego, California 92122

8910 Villa La Jolla Drive, La Jolla, California 92037

8939 Villa La Jolla Drive, La Jolla, California 92037

8950 Villa La Jolla Drive, La Jolla, California 92037

9333 Genesee Avenue, San Diego, California 92121

Sites That Are Part of UC San Diego Health, Hillcrest –

Fourth and Lewis Medical Offices, 330 Lewis Street, San Diego, California 92103

Medical Offices South, 4168 Front Street, San Diego, California 92103

140 Arbor Drive, San Diego, California 92103

410 Dickinson Street, San Diego, California 92103

[*]This list does not include outlying sites which are numerous and under continual development in varying constructs.

Appendix F: Buildings (All Sites with Location; Arranged in Chronological Order)

UC San Diego Medical Center, Hillcrest (1963)

Basic Sciences Building, La Jolla West Campus (1968) (Later Renamed Biomedical Sciences Building)

UC San Diego Medical Center Outpatient Center, Hillcrest (1977)

Clinical Teaching Facility, Hillcrest (1978)

Medical Teaching Facility, La Jolla West Campus (1978)

Theodore Gildred Cancer Center and Medical Library, Hillcrest (1981)

Center for Molecular Genetics, La Jolla West Campus (1987) (Later Renamed Center for Neural Circuits and Behavior)

Cellular and Molecular Medicine West, La Jolla West Campus (1990)

Sam and Rose Stein Clinical Research Building, La Jolla West Campus (1991)

Shiley Eye Center, La Jolla East Campus (1991) (Renamed Shiley Institute in 2015)

New Bed Tower, UC San Diego Medical Center, Hillcrest (1991)

John M and Sally B Thornton Hospital, La Jolla East Campus (1993)

Edith and William M Perlman Ambulatory Care Center, La Jolla East Campus (1993)

Bannister Family House, Hillcrest (1994)

Cellular and Molecular Medicine East, La Jolla West Campus (1995)

Keck Magnetic Resonance Imaging Facility, La Jolla West Campus (2002)

Leichtag Family Foundation Biomedical Research Facility, La Jolla West Campus (2004)

Biomedical Library Expansion, La Jolla West Campus (2004)

Joan and Irwin Jacobs Retina Center, La Jolla East Campus (2004)

Hamilton Glaucoma Center, La Jolla East Campus (2004)

John and Rebecca Moores Cancer Center, La Jolla East Campus (2005)

Radiation Oncology PET/CT Center, La Jolla East Campus (2009)

Rita Atkinson Residences, La Jolla West Campus (2010)

Sanford Consortium for Regenerative Medicine, La Jolla North Torrey Pines Road (2011)

Sulpizio Family Cardiovascular Center, La Jolla East Campus (2011)

Center for Advanced Laboratory Medicine, La Jolla Campus Point Drive (2011)

East Campus Office Building, La Jolla East Campus (2011)

T. Denny Sanford Medical Education and Telemedicine Building, La Jolla West Campus (2011)

Centralized Research Support Facility, La Jolla West Campus (2013)

J. Craig Venter Institute, La Jolla Village Drive (2013)

Health Sciences Biomedical Research Facility II, La Jolla West Campus (2014)

Altman Clinical and Translational Research Institute, La Jolla East Campus (2016)

Jacobs Medical Center, La Jolla East Campus (2016)

Koman Family Outpatient Pavilion, La Jolla East Campus (2018)

About the Author

David N. Bailey, M.D.

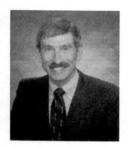

David N. Bailey received his Bachelor of Science degree in Chemistry "with high distinction"

from Indiana University and his Doctor of Medicine degree from Yale University, where he also

completed residency training in clinical pathology and subspecialty training in clinical chemistry.

He is board certified in clinical pathology with added qualification in chemical pathology

(American Board of Pathology). Dr. Bailey has served as Director of Clinical Laboratories at UC

San Diego Health System, Chair of the UC San Diego Department of Pathology, UC San Diego

Interim Vice Chancellor for Health Sciences and Dean of the School of Medicine, and UC Irvine

Vice Chancellor for Health Affairs and Dean of the School of Medicine. He also served as

President of the Academy of Clinical Laboratory Physicians and Scientists, President of the

California Association of Toxicologists, Secretary-Treasurer of the Association of Pathology

Chairs, and Secretary of the Association of Pathology Chairs Senior Fellows Group. He has

served on the editorial boards of *Clinical Chemistry*, *Journal of Analytical Toxicology*, and

American Journal of Clinical Pathology and on the Chemical Pathology Test Development and

Advisory Committee of the American Board of Pathology. Following retirement from UC Irvine

in 2009 he returned to UC San Diego as Distinguished Research Professor of Pathology and

Pharmacy, Vice Chair for Education and Academic Affairs in the Department of Pathology, and

Deputy Dean of the Skaggs School of Pharmacy and Pharmaceutical Sciences.

Made in the USA
San Bernardino, CA
23 January 2020